REVISION HANDBOOK OF CLINICAL HEMATOLOGY

A Short and Comprehensive Summary Note and Reference Guide of Hematology

Olivia Smith

AUTHOR'S ADDRESS

It is with deep sense of gratitude, humility, and fulfillment that I present this book to you esteemed reader.

This book, **Revision Handbook of Clinical Hematology,** is loaded with essential, high yield and clinically optimized information in all areas of Hematology including all sub-topics under Hematopoiesis, Anemias, Hemostasis, Blood transfusion and Hematological malignancies.

The book is a complex extract from standard texts of Hematology. It is carefully written in a friendly, easily comprehensible and logically sequential manner, using tables and illustrations that enhance easy understanding.

It simplifies the stepwise approach to accurate diagnosis of hematological disorders through history taking, physical examination and laboratory investigations.

I promise you will really enjoy studying Hematology using this book. If you did enjoy it, I will be very grateful if you would post a short review on Amazon. Thank you!!!

With Gratitude,
Dr Olivia Smith.

TABLE OF CONTENT

SECTION I: INTRODUCTION TO HEMATOLOGY

CHAPTER 1: HEMATOPOIESIS

- ▪ **Definition**
- − Hematopoiesis is the process of formation and development of cellular elements of the blood
- − The term hematopoiesis comprises the following:

- • **Erythropoiesis**: red blood cell formation
- • **Leukopoiesis**: granulocyte, monocyte and lymphocyte formation
- • **Thrombopoiesis**: platelet formation

- ❖ **Sites of hematopoiesis**

- ▪ **Intrauterine life (IUL)**
- - **Yolk sac:** this is the main site of hematopoiesis within the first 2 months of IUL
- - **Spleen and liver:** they take over within the 2nd and 7th months of IUL
- - **Bone marrow:** the most important site of blood cell formation from the 5th month of IUL and in the EUL

- ▪ **Extrauterine life (EUL)**
- • **In Infants**
- − The marrow of all bones is the site of hematopoiesis.

- • **In adulthood**
- − Only the marrow of membranous bones i.e. the vertebrae, ribs, sternum, skull, sacrum, and pelvis, and the proximal ends of femurs and humeri are involved in hematopoiesis

- Note especially that these are mainly the bones of the axial skeleton

❖ Forms of hematopoiesis

- During the intrauterine life, two forms of hematopoiesis occur; they include:
- Primitive hematopoiesis
- Definitive hematopoiesis

▪ Primitive hematopoiesis

- This is the formation of blood cells from the blood island of the extra-embryonic yolk sac.
- It continues till the 8th week in humans; red cells are the main blood cells produced.

▪ Definitive hematopoiesis

- This arises slightly later than the primitive hematopoiesis
- It begins in the splanchno-pleura or aorta-gonad-mesonephros of the developing embryo
- It continues throughout postnatal life; all blood cells are produced

CHAPTER 2: ERYTHROPOIESIS

- **Introduction**
- Due to the inability of erythrocytes to divide and replenish their own number, the old ruptured cells must be replaced by entirely new ones from the bone marrow

- **Definition**
- Erythropoiesis is a complex and finely regulated process whereby new red blood cells are generated for body needs.

- **Sites of Erythropoiesis**
- Intrauterine life: yolk sac, liver, spleen, bone marrow
- Extrauterine life: bone marrow

- **Rate of Erythropoiesis**
- About 1 billion (10^9) new red blood cells are generated daily
- Each erythropoietic cycle takes 7days (1 week)

- **Stages of Erythropoiesis**
- Pronormoblast (proerythroblast)
- Early normoblast (basophilic erythroblast)
- Intermediate normoblast (polychromatophilic erythroblast)
- Late normoblast (orthochromatic erythroblast)
- Reticulocyte

- Each stage is described below based on the cell size, cytoplasmic staining, hemoglobin concentration and nuclear changes.

- **Pronormoblast (proerythroblast)**
- This is the first recognisable erythrocyte precursor in the bone marrow
- The largest cell of the lineage
- Has a basophilic cytoplasm (due to abundance of ribosomes)
- Has a centrally placed nucleus containing nucleoli and slightly clumped chromatin
- It undergoes progressive series of cell divisions to give 4 basophilic erythroblasts.

- **Early normoblast (basophilic erythroblast)**
- This is smaller than the proerythroblast
- Has a basophilic cytoplasm (due to abundance of ribosomes)
- Has a smaller nucleus with a more clumped chromatin
- Hemoglobin synthesis has started
- Each of the cell divide to give a total of 8 polychromatophilic erythroblast

- **Intermediate normoblast (polychromatophilic erythroblast)**
- This is smaller than the early normoblast
- Its cytoplasm stains blue (due to ribosomal RNA) and pink (due to hemoglobin), hence its name
- The nucleus appears smaller with highly condensed chromatin
- It continues to synthesis hemoglobin
- It is the last precursor cell capable of mitosis
- Each divides to give a total of 16 orthochromatic erythroblasts

- **Late normoblast (orthochromatic erythroblast)**
- This is smaller than the polychromatic erythroblast
- It has an acidophilic (pink staining) cytoplasm, due to its high hemoglobin concentration

- The nucleus is small and pyknotic; thus incapable of mitosis
- Extrusion of the nucleus and other organelles from these cells convert them into reticulocytes

■ **Reticulocyte**
- This is slightly larger than the mature erythrocyte
- It contains some ribosomes which account for the little hemoglobin synthesis seen at this stage
- Clustering of the remnant ribosomes form a reticular network within the cell; hence its name
- It spends 1-2 days within the bone marrow and another 1-2 days in the peripheral blood

■ **Maturation**
- Final maturation of reticulocytes into a complete pink-staining, non-nucleated, biconcave disc erythrocyte takes place in the spleen.

❖ **Factors necessary for normal erythropoiesis**
● **Erythropoietin**
- A heavily glycosylated polypeptide of 165 aminoacids and molecular weight of 34 kDa.
- 90% is produced in the peritubular interstitial cells of the kidney, and the rest by the liver
- It acts on the bone marrow cells to stimulate erythropoiesis

● Vitamins - vitamin B12, folic acid (B9), pyridoxine (B6) etc.
● Other hormones – androgens, thyroid hormone, growth hormone etc.
● Iron (Fe)
● Trace elements – Copper, Zinc, Cobalt, Nickel etc.

- Protein (amino acids)

CHAPTER 3: HEMOGLOBIN (Hb)

- Since the main function of erythrocytes is to transport oxygen to the tissues and return carbon dioxide to the lungs, they require the presence of a specialized protein; called hemoglobin (Hb).

- **Each red cell contains about 640 million molecules of Hb, and each Hb molecule has a molecular weight of 68,000**

- **Types of hemoglobin in normal adult blood**
- Hemoglobin A_1 (HbA$_1$) – 96 to 98%
- Hemoglobin A_2 (HbA$_2$) – 1.5 to 3.2%
- Hemoglobin F (HbF) – 0.5 to 0.8 %

❖ **Hemoglobin Synthesis**

▪ **Sites of synthesis**
- Nucleus, mitochondria and cytoplasm of the erythroblasts

▪ **Stages of synthesis**
- Heme synthesis
- Globin synthesis
- Hemoglobin synthesis

▪ **Heme synthesis**
- The heme part of hemoglobin is synthesised within the mitochondria.
- Under the action of the enzyme; δ-aminolaevulinic acid (ALA) synthase and its coenzyme; pyridoxal phosphate (vitamin B6)

glycine is condensed with succinyl coenzyme A to form porphobilinogen.
- Porphobilinogen is progressively converted to uroporphyrinogen, then to coproporphyrinogen and eventually to protoporphyrin.
- Finally, protoporphyrin combines with ferrous iron (Fe^{2+}) supplied by circulating transferrin, to form heme.

- **Globin synthesis**
- The globin chain of hemoglobin is synthesised partly by the nucleus and the cytoplasm.
- Within the nucleus, the gene coding for globin chain lies on chromosomes 11 and 16.
- Following stimulation by erythropoietin, the genes are transcribed into messengerRNA (mRNA).
- The globin mRNA in turn enters the cytoplasm and attaches to cytoplasmic ribosomes.
- With the contribution of transfer and ribosomal RNA, the mRNA is translated into globin chains

- **Hemoglobin synthesis**
- The combination of heme and globin to form Hb ultimately takes place within the cytoplasm.
- Each molecule of heme combines with a globin chain to form a chain of hemoglobin (α, β, γ etc.)
- Four hemoglobin chains in turn combine to form a molecule of hemoglobin.

- **Genetic basis of globin chain synthesis**
- The gene coding for synthesis of globin chain of Hb lies on chromosomes 11 and 16.
- On each of the chromosomes, the genes occurs in clusters:

- Chromosome 11 - β,γ,δ and ε genes
- Chromosome 16 - α and ζ genes

— Each of the genes codes for a corresponding chain of hemoglobin during the embryonic, fetal and adult lives, depending on the form of Hb appropriate for that period.

— For example, in the embryo, and fetus, Gower 1, Portland, Gower 2 and fetal Hb dominate at different stages.

— In the extrauterine life, fetal Hb dominate for the first 3 to 6 months, after which it is replaced by adult HbA; when synthesis of the β-chain largely replace its γ-chain.

— Combination of the various globin chain to give the different forms of Hb is as follows:

- HbA1 - $\alpha_2\beta_2$ Gower 1 - $\zeta_2\varepsilon_2$
- HbA2 - $\alpha_2\delta_2$ Portland - $\zeta_2\gamma_2$
- HbF - $\alpha_2\gamma_2$ Gower 2 - $\alpha_2\varepsilon_2$

■ **Mechanism of action of hemoglobin**

— By virtue of the hemoglobin they possess, red cells are able to carry O_2 from the lungs to the tissue, and is able to return CO_2 from the tissue to the lungs

— As the Hb molecule loads and unloads O_2, the individual globin chains in the Hb molecule slide over each other, and the $\alpha_1\beta_1$ and $\alpha_2\beta_2$ contacts stabilize the molecule.

— Functionally, hemoglobin exists in two forms:
- Taut (T) form – in deoxygenated state
- Relaxed (R) form – in oxygenated state

✓ **Taut form**

— The taut form of Hb has low affinity for oxygen

— It is found at the tissue level and favours oxygen release to the tissue

- Factors such as low pH, high CO_2, and high 2, 3 DPG favours this form of Hb

✓ **Relaxed form**
- This is form of Hb has high affinity for oxygen
- It is found in the lungs and favours co-operative binding of oxygen to Hb molecule
- Factors such as high pH, low CO_2, and low 2, 3 DPG favours this form of Hb

• **Function of Fetal Hemoglobin**
- Hemoglobin F (HbF) has a higher affinity for oxygen than HbA_1; this is because HbF has γ-chain (which has no affinity for 2, 3 DPG)
- Thus at the placenta level where the partial pressure of oxygen (PO_2) is low, and the concentration of 2, 3 DPG is high; HbA_1 readily looses O_2 to HbF.
- Due to its higher affinity, HbF binds the O_2 and transport it to the fetal tissue for utilization.

CHAPTER 4 PLATELET

- ▪ **Introduction**
- — Platelets are small anucleated cells produced in the bone marrow by fragmentation of the cytoplasm of megakaryocytes.
- — Megakaryocytes are one of the largest cells in the body, produced within the bone marrow from their precursors; the megakaryoblasts
- — The megakaryoblasts are derived from the CFU-Meg of the CFU-$_{GEMM}$ of the PHSC

- ▪ **Thrombopoiesis**
- — Thrombopoiesis simply means the formation of blood platelets

- ● **Process of Thrombopoiesis**
- — The megakaryocyte once formed; mature by endomitotic synchronous replication (ESR)
- — ESR is a form of replication whereby there is DNA replication in the absence of nuclear or cytoplasmic division.
- — ESR causes the nuclear lobes to increase in multiples of two, per DNA replication i.e. 2n, 4n, 8n etc. with concurrent enlargement of the cytoplasmic volume.
- — Following maturation by ESR, the megakaryocyte develops into a highly branched network which produces invaginations of the plasma membrane called demarcation membranes.
- — Mature megakaryocytes are extremely large, with eccentrically placed single lobulated nucleus.
- — Platelets are eventually formed by fragmentation of the megakaryocyte cytoplasm.

- **Maturation**
- Each megakaryocyte gives rise to 1000 to 5000 platelets
- Following their release into the circulation, they are trapped in the spleen for about 36hrs, during which maturation occur.
- The entire process of thrombopoiesis takes about 10days
- Platelets have a life span of 7 to 10 days

- **Storage**
- About one-third of the marrow output of platelet is trapped within the spleen at any time; and about 90% of them can be trapped if there is splenomegaly.

- **Normal platelet count**
- Caucasian – 150 – 450 x 10^9/L
- African – 90 – 300 x 10^9/L

- **Regulator of thrombopoiesis**
- Thrombopoietin is the major regulator of platelet production.
- It is constitutively produced by the liver (about90%) and kidney
- They act on the c-Mpl receptor of the megakaryocyte to increase the number and rate of their maturation.

- **Structure of platelet**
- Platelets are extremely small, anucleated, discoid shaped cells.
- They are about 3.0 x 0.5 μm in diameter, with a mean volume 7-11 fL.

- **Platelet granules**
- The platelet contains 3 types of storage granules; namely:
- alpha- granules – 80%
- dense – granules

- lysosomes

— The α- granules contain: fibrinogen, fibronectin, von willebrand factor, selectin, plasminogen, α-2 antiplasmin, platelet derived growth factor, PDGF etc.
— The dense granules are less common and contain: ATP, ADP, serotonin, calcium, histamine, polyphosphates etc.
— Lysosomes contain hydrolytic enzymes e.g. esterases, lipases, nucleotidases, peptidases and phosphatises.

- **Platelet antigens**
— On their membranes, platelets also express ABO blood group antigens, as well as human leukocyte antigen (major histocompatiblity proteins)
— Note that, only class 1 MHC proteins are expressed by them

   ✓ *Roles of platelet in hemostasis are discussed in section 3*

CHAPTER 5:LEUKOCYTES

- **Leukopoiesis**: is the regulated formation of white blood cells i.e. granulocytes, monocyte and lymphocytes
- Granulocytes are mature granule-containing leukocytes; they include neutrophils, basophils, and eosinophils.
- Monocytes are large mononuclear phagocytic leukocyte found in blood, spleen, lymph nodes etc.
- Lymphocytes are small white cells formed in lymphatic tissue throughout the body e.g. lymph nodes, spleen, thymus, tonsils, Peyer patches, and sometimes in bone marrow

Development of Granulocytes
- This is also known as granulopoiesis
- Granulopoiesis proceeds through several stages:
- Myeloblast → Promyelocyte → Myelocyte → Metamyelocyte → Band (stab/juvenile) neutrophils → Neutrophil

Development of Monocytes
- Development of monocytes proceed through 5 stages:
- Monoblast/Myeloblast → Promonocyte → Monocyte → Immature macrophage → Mature macrophage

Development of Lymphocytes
- This is also known as lymphopoiesis

Process of lymphopoiesis
- During stem cell differentiation in the bone marrow; common lymphoid progenitor cells arise from the PHSC
- The common lymphoid progenitor cells differentiate into distinct lymphocyte types (B and T lymphocytes) and the natural killer cells.
- The B-cells remain within the bone marrow where they develop into mature B lymphocyte

- The T-cells migrate to the thymus for maturation
- Following maturation in the primary lymphoid organs (bone marrow and thymus) they migrate to the secondary lymphoid organs; the spleen, lymph node, peyers patches etc. where they survey for invading pathogens and/or tumor cells

- **Morphology and Function of Leukocytes**
- **Neutrophils**
- **Structure**
- Neutrophils are commonly referred to as polymorphonuclear leukocytes
- They constitute about 60 to 70% of total blood leukocyte
- They have a dense nucleus having 2 to 5 lobes
- Following their release from the bone marrow, they stay only for 12 hrs in the blood
- About 50% of them are seen in the circulating blood while the other 50% are found in the marginated pool, attached to blood vessel walls.
- After transmigrating to the tissue, they survive only for about 5days

- **Granules**
- Their granules are divided into two (primary and secondary) both of which are of lysosomal origin:
- Primary/azurophilic granules consisting of - myeloperoxidase, acid phosphatase, serine protease, elastase, defensin, bacterial permeability increasing protein (BPIP) etc.
- Secondary granules; consisting of: collagenase, lactoferrin, lysosyme, alkaline phosphatase etc.

- **Function**
- They are usually the first responders to microbial infection and acute inflammation
- They defend the body against bacterial and fungal infection

- **Eosinophil**
- **Structure**
- Eosinophils are similar to neutrophils except that their granules are coarser and stain more intensely red
- Their nucleus usually has 2 lobes but rarely exceeds 3
- Their bilobed nucleus appears like spectacle
- They stay longer in blood than neutrophils

- **Functions**
- They primarily deal with parasitic infections.
- They are also the predominant inflammatory cells in allergic reactions
- They defend against certain tumors
- They remove fibrin formed during inflammation

- **Basophil**
- **Structure**
- They have characteristic dark granules which overlie the nucleus
- Their nucleus may be bi- or trilobed but difficult to see (due to the granules)
- Their degranulation results from binding of IgE to their receptor, to release histamine and heparin

- **Function**
- They are chiefly responsible for allergic and anaphylactic reactions
- They also help in controlling parasitic infection

- Lymphocyte
- Structure
  - They are approximately the size of erythrocytes
  - Their nucleus is not lobulated; it stains deeply and eccentric in location
  - They are rarely granulated
  - They are of tree types: B-cell, T-cell and natural killer (NK) cells

- Function
  - B-cells produce antibodies against pathogens
  - CD4+ helper T-cells binds antigen presented by MHC II of antigen presenting cells (APC)
  - CD8+ cytotoxic cells bind antigens presented by MHC I of tumor or virus-infected cells
  - NK cells kill body cells that has lost MHC I or as become cancerous or viral-infected

- Monocytes
- Structure
  - They are larger than most other blood cells
  - They have abundant cytoplasm having many fine vacuoles that stains blue
  - Fine granules are often present
  - Their nucleus is large and indented with clumped chromatin
  - After spending 20 to 40hrs in the blood, they enter the tissue to become macrophages

- Function
  - They perform phagocytotic function in bacterial, parasitic, and fungal infection

23

SECTION II   ANEMIAS

CHAPTER 6: INTRODUCTION TO ANEMIAS

- **Introduction**
- Hematocrit a.k.a. packed cell volume (PCV) is defined as; the proportion of the volume of a blood sample that is red blood cells.

- **Red Cell Indices**
- Red cell indices are derivatives of blood tests that provide information about the hemoglobin content and size of red blood cells
- They are useful in elucidating the etiology of anemias; they include:
  - Mean corpuscular volume (MCV)
  - Mean corpuscular hemoglobin (MCH)
  - Mean corpuscular hemoglobin concentration (MCHC)

- **Mean corpuscular volume (MCV)**
- This is a measure of the average volume (i.e. size) of a red cell
- Its formula is PCV/RBC count
- It is measured in femtoLitre (fL); normal value is 80 – 95 fL
- It helps to determine whether a RBC is normocytic, macrocytic or microcytic

- **Mean corpuscular hemoglobin (MCH)**
- This is a measure of the average weight of Hb in a red cell
- The formula is HB conc/RBC count
- It is measured in pictogram (pg); normal value is 27 – 34 pg

- **Mean corpuscular hemoglobin concentration (MCHC)**
- This is a measure of the average concentration of Hb in a red cell

- Its formula is Hb conc/PCV
- It is measured in g/dL; normal value is 30 – 35 g/dL
- It helps to determine whether a RBC is normochromic, hyperchromic or hypochromic

- **Anemia**
- Anemia is defined as hemoglobin concentration below the value considered normal for the age, sex and race of an individual

- **Age**
- Children have a higher hemoglobin concentration and PCV than adults

- **Sex**
- Females have a lower Hb concentration and PCV than males of the same post-pubertal age; this is due to the effect of sex hormones; testosterone which stimulates erythropoiesis, and the monthly menstrual bleeding
- Normal HB concentration in male and female is as follows:
  - Male – 13.5 to 17.5 g/dL
  - Female – 11.5 to 15.5 g/dL
- Thus among adults, anemia may be defined as decreased Hb concentration below 13.5 g/dL in males and below 11.5 g/dL in females.

- **Race**
- The higher an area is located, the more the PCV of people residing there.
- For instance, Kenyans and Ethiopians, who reside at higher altitudes, usually have a PCV greater than that of a corresponding Americans.

- **Classification of anemia**
- Anemia can be classified based on two criteria:
  - Based on RBC morphology
  - Based on etiology

- **Based on RBC morphology (RBC indices)**
- This is the most useful and most acceptable classification criterion for therapeutic purpose, as it gives information about the primary defect causing the anemia
- Using this criterion, anemia is classified as:
  - Hypochromic anemia
  - Microcytic anemia
  - Macrocytic anemia
  - Normocytic normochromic anemia

- **Hypochromic anemia**
- Anemia characterised by a reduction in the Hb concentration of red cell in the peripheral blood.
- The central area of pallor of the RBC is > one-third of its diameter
- MCH is < 27pg, and MCHC is <30g/dL

Causes
- Iron deficiency anemia – most common
- Thalassemia
- Lead poisoning
- Sideroblastic anemia
- Anemia of chronic disorder

- **Microcytic anemia**
- Anemia characterised by presence of small-sized RBC (microcytes) in the peripheral blood
- MCH is < 27pg, and MCV is <80fL

- Microcytic and hypochromic anemia usually occur together; thus, are collectively referred to as microcytic hypochromic anemia

Causes
- Sideroblastic anemia
- Iron deficiency anemia
- hereditary spherocytosis
- autoimmune hemolytic anemia

- **Macrocytic anemia**
- Anemia characterised by presence of larger than normal RBC in the peripheral blood
- They lack the usual central area of pallor of normal RBCs
- MCV is > 95fL and MCH is > 34pg

Causes
- Aplastic anemia
- Megaloblastic anemia
- Chronic blood loss
- Alcohol abuse
- Cytotoxic drugs e.g. methotrexate

- **Normocytic normochromic anemia**
- Anemia characterised by presence of normal sized RBC containing normal Hb concentration in the peripheral blood.
- Anemia here is due to a decrease in total RBC count; as all RBC indices are normal

Causes
- Anemia of chronic disorder
- Renal failure
- Acute blood loss
- Bone marrow failure

- **Based on Etiology**
- Based on the causative agent, anemia can be broadly classified as:

- **Anemia due to blood loss**
- Acute blood loss
- Chronic blood loss

- **Anemia due to reduced production of RBC**
- Nutrient deficiency (Iron, folate, VitB$_{12}$)
- Hypoproliferative marrow

- **Anemia due to excessive destruction or consumption of RBCs**
- Hemolytic anemia
- Hypersplenism
- Disseminated intravascular coagulation (DIC)

✓ *Details of the above will be the subject of discussion in subsequent chapters*

Clinical features of anemia

Symptoms of anemia	Signs of anemia
− Weakness / undue tiredness	− Palor
− Easy fatigability	− Tachycardia
− Intermittent claudication	− Systolic murmur
− Palpitation	− Bounding pulse
− Headache	
− Lethargy	
− Confusion	

❖ Laboratory investigation of Anemia

▪ General tests

● **Peripheral blood smear**
- To know the RBC size (normocytic, macrocytic or microcytic)
- To know the Hb conc (normochromic, hyperchromic or hypochromic)

● **Bone marrow aspiration and cytology**
- To rule out haematological malignancy and metastasis

● **Reticulocyte count**
- To differentiate marrow failure (count is low) from hemolytic anemia (count is high)

● **Special tests**
- Iron staining
- Serum ferritin
- Red cell and serum folate estimation
- Hb electrophoresis
- DNA analysis

▪ Treatment of anemia
- Blood transfusion (if symptomatic or severe)
- Treat the underlying cause

CHAPTER 7: HEMOLYTIC ANEMIAS

- **Introduction**
- Hemolytic anemias are a group of disorders characterised by accelerated red cell destruction
- Thus, it is characterised by shortened survival of mature erythrocytes
- It occurs due to inability of the bone marrow to cope with the rate at which erythrocytes are destroyed, but not due to impaired ability of the bone marrow to respond.

- **Normal red destruction**
- Normally, red cell destruction usually occurs after a mean life span of 100 to 120 days
- They are destroyed by macrophages of the reticuloendothelial system

- **Break down products of erythrocyte**
- Following the destruction of red cells; iron, globin and protoporphyrin are released into the circulation
- The iron is recirculated via plasma transferrin to bone marrow erythroblasts
- The globin chains are broken down to amino acids; which are reutilized for general protein synthesis
- The protoporphyrin is broken down to bilirubin (this accounts for the appearance of jaundice in patient with hemolytic anemia)

- **Haptoglobins**
- Haptoglobin is a 100 KDa, α_2 – globulin protein present in normal plasma
- It irreversibly binds free hemoglobin in plasma to form hemoglobin – Haptoglobin complex

- This complex is promptly removed by the liver; thus prevents loss of free hemoglobin in the urine
- Haptoglobin levels are decreased by increased hemolysis, and increased by acute conditions such as infection, burn, tissue destruction etc.

❖ Classification of hemolytic anemias

- Hemolytic anemias (HA) can be classified in several ways, depending on whether:
  - It was inherited or acquired
  - The hemolysis is due to an intrinsic or extrinsic RBC defect
  - The hemolysis occur extravascularly or intravascularly

- Note that; hereditary HA are usually the result of an intrinsic red cell defect, while acquired HA are usually the result of an extrinsic red cell defect.
- However, an exception to the above statement is seen in paroxysmal nocturnal hemoglobinuria (PNH) where an acquired HA results from an intrinsic red cell defect

▪ Hereditary or intrinsic hemolytic anemia

- This may occur due to any of the following red cell defects, each of which is followed by examples of the specific diseases caused by the defect:

● **Defects in hemoglobin synthesis (hemoglobinopathies)**
- Thalassemia
- Sickle cell disease
- Hemoglobin C disease
- Unstable hemoglobin

● **Defects of red cell membrane synthesis**
- Hereditary spherocytosis
- Hereditary elliptocytosis

- **Defects of red cell metabolism**
- **Glucose-6-phosphate dehydrogenase (G6PD) deficiency**
- **Pyruvate kinase deficiency**

- **Acquired or extrinsic hemolytic anemia**
  - These are hemolytic anemia resulting from non-hereditary or extrinsic red cell defects, except of course in PNH; they include:

- **Immune mediated hemolytic anemia**
  - Autoimmune hemolytic anemia
  - Alloimmune hemolytic anemia

- **Non-immune mediated hemolytic anemia**
  - Drugs - e.g. ribavirin
  - Toxins - e.g. snake venom
  - Infections - e.g. malaria, babesiosis
  - Red cell fragmentation syndromes
  - March hemoglobinuria
  - Paroxysmal nocturnal hemoglobinuria
  - Liver disorders

- **Clinical features of hemolytic anemias**
  - General symptoms and signs of anemia
  - Splenomegaly
  - Excess urobilinogen excretion
  - Pigment (bilirubin) gallstone

- **Laboratory findings in hemolytic anemias**
  - The laboratory findings are conveniently divided into three groups:

- **Features of increased red cell break down**
  - Raised serum bilirubin

- Increased urine urobilinogen
- Increased fecal stercobilinogen
- Low/absent serum haptoglobins

- **Features of increased red cell production**
- Reticulocytosis
- Hyperplasia of marrow erythroid cells

- **Features of malformed red cells**
- Abnormal red cell morphology e.g. microspherocytes, elliptocytes etc
- Increased osmotic fragility
- Shortened red cell survival

- **Treatment of hemolytic anemia**
- Blood transfusion (if indicated)
- Treat the underlying cause

CHAPTER 8: HEMOGLOBINOPATHIES

- **Introduction**
- Hemoglobinopathies are genetic disorders of hemoglobin
- They are inherited hematological diseases, whereby a mutant globin gene is inherited from both parents who, though are generally healthy, are carriers
- Thus hemoglobinopathies are autosomal recessive disorders

- **Definition**
- Hemoglobinopathies are inherited, quantitative or qualitative defect in either the α or β chain of hemoglobin

- **Epidemiology**
- Hemoglobinopathies are the most prevalent single gene disorders world-wide
- They affect approximately 7% of the world's population, especially people of the tropics and subtropics

- **Classification of hemoglobinopathies**
- Broadly, hemoglobinopathies are classified into two:

- **Quantitative hemoglobinopathies**
- Thalassemias

- **Qualitative / structural hemoglobinopathies**
- Sickle cell disorder
- Sickle cell trait
- Hemoglobin C disease
- Hemoglobin D disease
- Hemoglobin E disease

❖ THALASSEMIAS

▪ Introduction

– Thalassemias are a heterogeneous group of genetic disorders characterised by a reduced synthesis of α or β chain of hemoglobin, due to a relative or an absolute deficiency in the number of coding genes

▪ Types

– Depending on the affected globin chain, thalassemias can be divided into two:
  • Alpha thalassemia
  • Beta thalassemia

▪ **Alpha Thalassemia**

• Basis

– Normally, there are four copies of the α - globin genes; two of which are inherited from each parent
– The four genes code for the two α-chains of hemoglobin
– Alpha thalassemia occurs when there is a complete or partial deletion of the four genes
– Note that the usual genetic lesion in alpha thalassemia is gene deletion
– The mode of inheritance is autosomal recessive

• Epidemiology

– Alpha thalassemia is more common in the Far East, south–east Asia, Middle East, china etc.
– Fortunately, these areas are malaria-endemic zones and the carrier state of thalassemia affords some protection against it

- **Classification**
- Based on the number genes deleted or inactivated among the four genes, alpha thalassemia can be classified into four:
  - Alpha thalassemia major
  - Hemoglobin H – disease
  - Alpha thalassemia minor
  - Silent carriers
- Note that both alpha thalassemia minor and silent carriers are called alpha thalassemia trait

- **Alpha thalassemia major**
- This condition results from loss of all four α–globin genes
- Since there is complete suppression of α–chain synthesis, this condition is not compatible with life and leads to inutero fetal death (hydrops fetalis)

- **Hemoglobin H disease**
- This condition results from loss of three (of the four) α–globin genes
- Here, α-chain synthesis is powered by only one gene; causing a great reduction in its level, and leaves the β - chain with nothing to pair with.
- The β-chain then begin to associate in groups of four; to produce abnormal hemoglobin called hemoglobin H.
- Inutero, the patient has hemoglobin Barts (Hb Barts); an Hb with four γ-chains (γ_4)
- The patient show severe microcytic, hypochromic anemia with splenomegaly
- Patient requires blood transfusion for survival

- **Alpha thalassemia minor**
- This condition results from loss of two α–globin genes

- They are usually asymptomatic; however, a very mild microcytic hypochromic anemia may be seen on routine blood testing
- This condition may be misdiagnosed as iron deficiency anemia; however, iron therapy does not correct the anemia

- **Silent carriers**
- This condition results from loss of one α–globin genes
- Since this condition is very difficult to detect, and affected individuals are usually normal; they are called silent carriers

- **Diagnosis**
- **α/β-globin chain synthesis study**
- The normal hemoglobin $\alpha : \beta$ of 1 to 1 is reduced in alpha thalassemia

- **Beta Thalassemia**
- **Basis**
- Normally, there are two copies of the β - globin genes; one of which is inherited from each parent
- The two β- globin genes code for the two β - chains of hemoglobin
- Beta thalassemia occurs when there is a complete or partial deletion of the two genes
- Note that the usual genetic lesion in beta thalassemia is **point mutation**
- The mode of inheritance is autosomal recessive

- **Epidemiology**
- Beta thalassemia is more common in the Mediterranean region.

- **Classification**
- Beta thalassemia is classified into three:
  - Beta thalassemia major
  - Beta thalassemia intermedia
  - Beta thalassemia minor

- **Beta thalassemia major**
- This condition results due to loss of both β-globin genes
- Hence, the hemoglobin produced after 3 to 6 month of birth lacks the β-chains
- Affected children are usually normal at birth; they develop symptoms and signs within the first 2 years of life, as there are no β - chains to replace the declining γ - chains
- The excess α-chains precipitate in erythroblasts and erythrocytes, causing their rapid hemolysis.
- The rapid red cell destruction results in a severe anemia called Cooley's anemia
- Patient often requires a life-long transfusion to survive.

- **Clinical features**
- **Severe anemia:** apparent at 3 to 6 month of age
- **Hepatosplenomegaly:** due to excessive red cell destruction, extra-medullary hemopoiesis etc.
- Intense marrow hyperplasia causing bone expansion – hair-on-end appearance of the skull is seen on X-ray.
- **Iron overload:** leading to organ damage, slately grey appearance of the skin etc
- **Infections:** by organisms including pneumococcus, hemophilus, meningococcus, and yersinia (especially in iron overload)
- **Osteoporosis:** in well-transfused patients

- Laboratory diagnosis
- **Peripheral blood smear**
  - Severe hypochromic microcytic anemia
  - Reticulocytosis, with normoblast and target cells
  - Basophilic stippling (presence of basophilic granules in the erythrocyte cytoplasm)

- **Hemoglobin electrophoresis**
  - Almost complete absence of HbA_1 with almost all circulating hemoglobin being HbF
  - HbA_2 level may be normal, low or slightly raised

- **α/β-globin chain synthesis study**
  - The normal hemoglobin $\alpha : \beta$ of 1 to 1 is increased in beta thalassemia

- **Assessment of patient iron status**
  - Serum ferritin
  - Serum iron and iron binding capacity

- Management
  - Regular blood transfusions- to maintain the Hb concentration at > 10 g/L at all times
  - Regular folic acid supplement
  - Iron chelation therapy – using IV deferoxamine or oral deferiprone
  - Vitamin C supplement – 200mg/day
  - Splenectomy - done after patient is older than 6yrs
  - Endocrine therapy – as replacement in end-organ damage
  - Immunization – against hepatitis B and C
  - Allogeneic bone marrow transplantation – definitive treatment

- **Beta – thalassemia minor**
- This condition is due to loss of one (of the two) β-globin gene
- Though this condition is common, it is usually asymptomatic; but a very mild microcytic hypochromic anemia may be seen on routine blood testing
- This condition as well may be misdiagnosed as iron deficiency anemia; however, iron therapy does not correct the anemia

- **Beta – thalassemia intermedia**
- As in β-thalassemia major, this condition result from loss of both β - globin genes; however, their clinical severity makes the difference
- The clinical severity of β–thalassemia intermedia lies between the mild symptoms of β-thalassemia minor and the severe manifestation of β–thalassemia major
- Based on the type of mutation involved, anemia can be mild or severe; however, many intermedia patients do not require transfusion for survival

- **Clinical feature**
- Bone deformities
- Hepatosplenomegaly
- Extramedullary hemopoiesis
- Features of iron overload

- ❖ **SICKLE CELL DISORDER**

- ▪ **Introduction**
- Sickle cell disorders (SCD) are a heterogeneous group of genetic disease of hemoglobin characterised by the inheritance of an abnormal "sickle" β-globin gene with another abnormal β-globin gene

- It is associated with production of fragile sickle-shaped erythrocytes, prone to untimely hemolysis

- **Definition**
- SCD is the inheritance of two abnormal forms of hemoglobin with at least one being hemoglobin S

- **Variants of hemoglobin**
- These are mutant forms of hemoglobin present in a population
- More than 500 Hb variants exist, though most are rarely encountered
- Clinically important Hb variants are as follows; in other of severity:
  - Hb SS – sickle cell anemia
  - Hb SC – sickle cell - hemoglobin C disease
  - Hb SD – sickle cell - hemoglobin D disease
  - Hb S-βthal – sickle cell - thalassemia disease

❖ SICKLE CELL ANEMIA (Hb SS)

- **Definition**
- Sickle cell anemia is a hematological disorder due to the homozygous inheritance of the sickle hemoglobin gene, resulting in sickling of erythrocytes in deoxygenated states manifesting ultimately in a chronic hemolytic anemia.

- **Epidemiology**
- Sickle cell anemia is widespread among West Africans (1 in 4 people)
- Nigeria has the highest cohort of SCA in Africa (about 2% of the population)
- It occur with lower frequency in the Mediterranean basin, Saudi Arabia, and parts of India

- As the carrier state (Hb AS) affords some protection against malaria, it tends to be more prevalent in malaria-endemic zones
- Note however that the homozygote state of this disease (Hb SS) gives no such protection, and in fact, the patient suffers more severe attacks of malaria

- **Molecular basis of SCA**
- The sickle gene mutation is due to the substitution of a single nucleotide; adenine by thymine in the second nucleotide of the 6th codon of the β-globin gene
- The nucleotide substitution results in the substitution of the amino acid; glutamic acid by valine at position 6 of the β-globin chain

	6th Codon of β-globin gene	Amino acid
Normal β-globin chain	GAG	Glutamic acid
Sickle β-globin chain	GTG	valine

- **Pathophysiology of SCA**
- The central problem of the Hb S is its tendency to become insoluble and crystallize in areas of low oxygen tension; as it contains the hydrophobic valine instead of the hydrophilic glutamic acid
- Initially, while in the deoxygenated state, RBCs assume the rigid sickle shape (sickling) due to Hb crystallisation; however following re-oxygenation, they return to their normal biconcave disc shape (unsickling)
- Ultimately, the repeated Sickling and unsickling of the cells, results in loss of membrane flexibility, causing occlusion of small blood vessels by entangled sickle erythrocytes.

- Loss of flexibility of the RBC membrane drastically shortens their survival, leading to a chronic hemolytic anemia
- Occlusion of small blood vessels causes sluggish blood flow (vascular stasis) resulting in ischemia or infarction of end organs
- In an attempt to compensate for the chronic anemia, bone marrow hyperplasia occur, resulting in high reticulocyte and nucleated erythrocyte count, as well as elevated leukocyte and platelet count
- The erythrocyte life span in sickle cell patient is shortened to as low as 15 to 25 days; average of 17 days

- Haplotypes of sickle cell gene
- Haplotype is a group of genes an individual inherits together from a single parent
- In relation to the β-globin gene; there are variations in structure of the DNA surrounding the gene locus among different population
- This account for the variability in clinical presentation of the diseases in different regions
- These variations in structure of the DNA surrounding the β-globin gene locus are known as haplotypes of sickle cell gene
- The haplotypes are named after the places where they were first described; they include:
    - Asian
    - Senegal
    - Bantu
    - Benin

- Clinical features of SCA
- Bone
- Dactylitis (hand and foot syndrome)

- Earliest clinical manifestation in sicklers
- Occurs between 6 and 18month of life
- Characterized by frequent bone pain and tenderness; affecting the limbs, ribs and vertebrae

- Bossing of the skull
- Bone marrow embolisation
- Multiple sited osteomylitis

- **Eye**
- Pallor
- Jaundice (persistent or recurrent)

- **Growth and development**
- Patient appear to be small for his age
- Delayed puberty

- **Spleen**
- Acute splenic sequestration (usually in children < 5yrs)
- On account of the above, spleen suffers repeated infarctions, which ultimately lead to autosplenectomy

- **Liver**
- Hepatomegaly
- Obstructive jaundice (due to gall stone)
- Acute hepatic sequestration

- **Urogenital system**
- Hyposthenuria (inability to form urine of high osmolality)
- Hematuria
- Renal papillary necrosis
- Renal failure
- Priampism (persistent, painful, purposeless penile erection)

- **Gall bladder**
- Bilirubin gallstone
- Cholecystitis

- **Laboratory Diagnosis SCA**
- **Peripheral blood smear**
- Presence of sickle cells and target cells
- Polychromasia in large RBCs
- Presence of Howell-jolly bodies (remnants of nuclear chromatin in the RBCs); a feature of splenic atrophy)

- **Sickling test**
- This is done by reducing the oxygen tension around the erythrocyte (using 2% sodium metabisulfite or sodium dithionite) and checking for sickling of the erythrocytes.
- This test detects sickle cell, but does not differentiate homozygote (Hb SS) from heterozygote state (Hb AS)

- **Solubility test**
- This works on the principle that Hb S is much less soluble than normal Hb
- It distinguishes homozygote (Hb SS) from heterozygote state (Hb AS) but does not distinguish heterozygote state (Hb AS) from doubly heterozygote state (Hb SC)

- **Hb electrophoresis**
- This separates different hemoglobin proteins based on their electric charge in solution
- There are two main types of Hb electrophoresis:

- **Cellulose acetate membrane electrophoresis**
- This is the recommended method; as it is easier and faster to perform; though final diagnosis cannot be said to have been reached using this method
- It is done at alkaline pH (8.6)

- **Citrate Agar electrophoresis**
- This is more difficult and time consuming; however it clearly differentiate Hb F, A_2, S, C and D
- it is done at acidic pH (6.1)

- **Prenatal diagnosis**
- Chorionic villous sampling; done at first trimester
- Amniocentesis; done at second trimester

❖ **Complications of SCA**
- Complications of sickle cell anemia can be classified as:
- Acute complications (crisis)
- Chronic complications

▪ **Acute complications (crisis)**
- These are essentially what we refer to as crisis
- There are four main types of sickle cell crisis:
- Vasoocclussive crisis
- Hyperhemolytic crisis
- Sequestration crisis
- Aplastic crisis

- **Vasoocclussive crisis**
- This is caused by occlusion of the small blood vessels (supplying end organs) by sickled erythrocyte; resulting in painful or painless ischemia or infarction of the organs; as shown in table 8.1

Painful vasoocclussive crisis	Painless vasoocclussive crisis
– Bone pain – Abdominal pain – Priampism – Acute chest syndrome	– Hematuria – Cerebrovascular disease

- **Hyperhemolytic crisis**
- This is characterised by acute increase in red cell destruction
- It is a life threatening condition leading to rapid drop in steady state PCV, and appearance or worsening of jaundice
- It is usually secondary to dehydration, stress, extremes of temperature, pregnancy, infection e.g. malaria etc.

- **Sequestration crisis**
- This caused by the sudden pooling of blood in visceral organs such as spleen (in children < 5) liver and mesentery

- **Aplastic crisis**
- This most commonly found among children
- A transient condition caused by infection of bone marrow erythroblast by parvovirus B19
- It is a self limiting condition, though may be life threatening

- **Chronic complications**
- **Skeletal system**
- Chronic osteomyelitis
- Avascular necrosis of the head of femur and humerus

- **Skin: Chronic leg ulcer**
- **Liver**
- Chronic viral hepatitis (due to repeated transfusion)
- Hemosiderosis (due to repeated transfusion)
- Gall stone (due to super-saturation of bile)

— Cholecystitis

- **Infection**

— By encapsulated organisms (pneumococcus, hemophilus, meningococcus etc.)

— Transfusion transmissible infections such as: human immunodeficiency virus (HIV) cytomegalovirus, hepatitis B and C etc.

- **Hypersplenism**

— Characterised by pancytopenia, and hypercellularity of the bone marrow

❖ **Management of SCA**

- **Objectives of management**

— To provide accurate diagnosis

— To maintain steady state of health

— To prevent and treat complication

— To give relevant health education and genetic counselling to the family and relatives

— To promote positive self image in them

- **Supportive**

— Heptavalent pneumococcal vaccine in children

— Hepatitis B vaccine

— Penicillin prophylaxis until age 5

— Periodic ophthalmic examination

— Folic acid supplement

— Paludrine (proguanil) as malaria prophylaxis

- ▪ Definitive
- **For painful crisis**
  - Rest
  - Rehydration
  - Analgesics
  - Oxygen supplement (if SPO_2 is low)

- **Exchange blood transfusion; for**
  - Stroke
  - Priampism
  - Acute chest syndrome
  - Intractable bone pain

- **Anti-sickling drugs**
  - Hydroxyurea (works by increasing HbF level)
  - Butyrate compound

- **Bone marrow transplantation**
  - Curative

Prevention

- Genetic counselling for families with sickle cell disorder

CHAPTER 9: DISORDERS OF RED CELL MEMBRANE SYNTHESIS

- **Normal red cell membrane**
- The normal red cell membrane is composed of:
  - Protein – 50%
  - Lipid – 40%
  - Carbohydrate – 10%

- **Lipids**
- The lipid portion (40%) is composed of the following:
  - Phospholipids – 60%
  - Neutral lipid – 30%
  - Glycolipids – 10%

- The outer leaflet of the RBC membrane consist mainly of phosphatidylcholine (lecithin) and sphingomyelin
- The inner leaflet consist mainly of phosphatidylethanolamine (cephalin) and phosphatidylserine
- The hydrophobic fatty acid portion points inwards, while the hydrophilic phosphate portion point outwards on both sides of the membrane i.e. towards the intracellular and extracellular fluid

- **Proteins**
- The protein portion (50%) can be structurally divided into two types:
  - Integral proteins – 60 – 80%
  - Peripheral protein – 20 – 40%

- The integral proteins span the entire membrane and provide channels connecting the plasma to the cytosol
- The cytosolic domain of these integral proteins interacts with each other and with the cytoskeleton of the red cell.

- Based on the above interaction, integral proteins can be classified into two forms: vertical and horizontal connections.
- Integral proteins linking the plasma surface of the membrane to the cytoskeleton are referred to as vertical connections; they include: β-spectrin, Band 3, Ankyrin and Protein 4.2

- Integral proteins making up the inner network of the membrane are referred to as horizontal connections; they include: α-spectrin, β-spectrin, Ankyrin, Protein 4.1 and Actin

- **Carbohydrates**
- The carbohydrates are composed of chains of monosaccharides, the majority of which are hexoses
- They occur only on the external surface of the membrane; not as free molecules, but complexed with proteins and lipids to form glycoproteins and glycolipids respectively

- **Classification of red cell membrane defects**
- **Genetic or intrinsic defect**
- Hereditary spherocytosis
- Hereditary elliptocytosis
- Hereditary pyropoikilocytosis
- South-East Asian ovalocytosis
- Hereditary stomatocytosis

- **Acquired or extrinsic defect**
- Acanthocytosis

- ✓ One notable exception is paroxysmal nocturnal hemoglobinuria (PNH) where an intrinsic defect is acquired as a result of somatic mutation.

❖ HEREDITARY SPHEROCYTOSIS

- **Introduction**
- Hereditary spherocytosis is a genetically determined hemolytic anemia characterized by the presence of spherical shaped red cells, called spherocytes, in plasma

- **Mode of inheritance**
- Usually autosomal dominant
- Rarely autosomal recessive

- **Etiology**
- It is usually caused by defects in the proteins involved in the vertical connections of the red cell membrane
- About 60% result from defect in the ankyrin-spectrin complex
- Another 25% involve deficiency of band 3 protein; the anion channel
- Abnormalities of protein 4.2 has also been described

- **Pathophysiology**
- The bone marrow produces normal biconcave disc shaped erythrocytes
- However, unsupported part of the membrane are lost over time and the cells become increasingly spherical
- Because the spherocytes are unable to manoeuvre through the splenic microvasculature, they rupture and die prematurely

- **Characteristics of spherocytes**
- They are spherical in shape
- Their diameter and surface area are reduced, but their volume remain the same
- They lack the central area of pallor typical of normal erythrocytes

— They stain more densely than normal erythrocyte

- **Clinical features**
— Chronic anemia
— Mild jaundice
— Increased osmotic fragility of erythrocytes
— Splenomegaly (rarely marked)
— Reticulocytosis
— Features of hemolytic anemia

- **Diagnosis**
— MCHC is increased
— MCV is decreased
— DNA analysis can be used to identify the defective gene or its product
— Increased osmotic fragility red cells
— Direct antiglobulin test; if normal rules out autoimmune causes of hemolysis

- **Treatment**
- **Blood transfusion**
— No transfusion is required in patients with well compensated hemolysis
— Transfusion is required in patients with severe hemolytic anemia

- **Cholecystectomy**
— In patients with recurrent cholecystitis

- **Splenectomy**
— In patients with severe anemia

❖ PAROXYSMAL NOCTURNAL HEMOGLOBINURIA (PNH)

- **Introduction**
- PNH is a rare, acquired, chronic disorder of hematopoietic stem cells characterized by chronic hemolytic anemia, thrombotic episodes and often pancytopenia

- **Distribution and epidemiology**
- PNH is a rare disorder with prevalence of 1 in 100,000
- It occurs in both children and adult with no apparent familial predisposition
- It occurs more frequently in South-East Asia and the Far East

- **Etiology**
- The primary defect in PNH is decreased synthesis of glycosylphosphatidyl inositol (GPI) anchor; a structure which attaches several proteins to the cell membrane

- **Genetic basis**
- PNH occurs due to a somatic mutation in the gene coding for phosphatidyl inositol glycan protein A (PIG-A); the gene is located on the short arm of X-chromosome

- **Pathophysiology**
- PIG-A is a protein essential for the synthesis of glycosylphosphatidyl inositol (GPI) anchor.
- GPI anchor are proteins whose function is to attach membrane-proteins to the membrane
- Thus, circulating erythrocytes derived from the mutated clone are deficient in the GPI-linked proteins, especially CD55 and CD 59:
  - ✓ CD55 - decay accelerating factor (DAF)
  - ✓ CD59 - membrane inhibitor of reactive lysis (MIRL)
- The absence of these proteins, both of which are regulators of compliment activation on the surface of the circulating red

cells, makes the red cells especially prone to hemolysis by the compliment system.
- The above in turn leads to a chronic intravascular hemolysis

- **Clinical features**
- **Hemoglobinuria**
- Passage of red or brownish urine on rising from sleep; regardless of the time of the day
- It may due to lowered blood pressure during sleep
- Infection, surgery, injection of contrast dye and strenuous exercise may as well trigger it

- **Hemosiderinuria**
- Loss of iron in urine, in form of hemosoderin and hemoglobin
- It is a constant feature and may result in iron deficiency anemia; worsening the background hemolytic anemia

- **Thrombosis**
- This is another main feature of PNH, though of obscure reason
- Venous thrombosis is the most frequent clinical manifestation of PNH
- Patient may develop recurrent hepatic vein thrombosis (Budd-chiari syndrome)

- **Chronic hemolysis**
- Features of anemia such as; weakness, pallor, and dyspnea are common
- Splenomegaly (moderate)

- **Bleeding**
- Due to thrombocytopenia (t vary from mild to severe)

- **Pregnancy**
- PNH may result in abortion as well as venous thromboembolism in pregnancy

- **Renal manifestation**
- Hyposthenuria
- Abnormal tubular function and declining creatinine clearance
- Hypertension (occasionally)
- Radiological findings of enlarged kidneys, cortical infarct, cortical thinning and papillary necrosis
- Acute or chronic renal failure may occur

- **Neurological manifestation**
- Venous sinus thrombosis may causes severe headache or eye ache
- Cerebral venous thrombosis is uncommon but fatal

- **Bone Marrow**
- Bone marrow aplasia and often frank aplastic anemia may occur

- **Diagnosis**
- **Flow cytometry**
- This is the gold standard of diagnosing PNH
- It is used to demonstrate the loss of expression of GPI-linked protein (DAF/CD55 and MIRL/CD59) while the red cells are suspended in fluid under a light focus

- **Ham test**
- Demonstrates the lysis of red cells in serum at low pH
- Has largely been replaced by flow cytometry

* **Treatment**
- Transfusion of washed red cells (to avoid transfusing compliment proteins)
- Iron therapy
- Steroid therapy
- Long term anticoagulant therapy e.g. warfarin
- Erythropoietin therapy

* **Eculizumab**
- A humanized antibody against compliment C5 which inhibit the activation of terminal component of compliment
- Thus reduces hemolysis and transfusion requirement

- Allogeneic stem cell transplantation is definitive
- Suppression of PNH cells with 6 mercaptopurine
- Cyclosporine in combination with granulocyte-colony stimulating factor (G-CSF) has been found useful

CHAPTER 10: DEFECTS OF RED CELL METABOLISM

- **Introduction**
- Mature erythrocytes are anucleate; thereby incapable of cell division, devoid of ribosomes; thereby incapable of protein synthesis, and lack mitochondria; thereby in capable of oxidative phosphorylation.
- In spite of all these limitations, they still survive 100 - 120 days! in the circulation and effectively deliver oxygen to peripheral tissue

- **Metabolism of glucose**
- Glucose is the main metabolic substrate of red blood cell, and it is metabolised by two main pathways:
- Glycolytic (energy-producing) pathway - > 90%
- Hexose mono-phosphate (protective) pathway – 5-10%

- **Role of Glycolytic pathway**
- The glycolytic pathway has three major end-products: ATP, NADH and 2, 3 DPG
- ATP is necessary for proper functioning of ATP-dependent membrane pumps; thus helps in maintaining cation homeostasis and membrane pliability in the red cells
- NADH is a cofactor essential for reduction of methemoglobin (Fe^{3+}) to Fe^{2+}
- 2, 3 DPG helps mediates binding of oxygen to hemoglobin, thereby facilitating the release of oxygen to the tissue.

- **Role of Hexose mono-phosphate (protective) pathway**
- The HMP shunt is the only source of NADPH in the erythrocyte
- NADPH is an important co-factor essential for the preservation and regeneration of reduced glutathione (GSH)
- Reduced glutathione (GSH) functions as an intracellular reducing agent that protects cells against oxidant injury

❖ GLUCOSE-6-PHOSPHATE DEHYDROGENASE (G6PD) DEFICIENCY

- **Introduction**
- G6PD deficiency is an inherited metabolic disorder, characterised by abnormally low level of the enzyme glucose-6-phosphate dehydrogenase (G6PD) in the body, especially in the red blood cells
- This disorder may result in hemolytic anemia because it predisposes to massive destruction of red cells following exposure to certain medications, food or infection

- **Normal function of G6PD and Pathophysiology of G6PD deficiency**
- G6PD is an important enzyme of the Hexose monophosphate shunt (pentose phosphate pathway)
- It catalyzes the oxidation of glucose-6-phosphate to 6-phosphogluconolactone, during which NADP is reduced to NADPH
- NADPH is required in the red cell for the formation of reduced glutathione (GSH)
- As free radicals readily oxidize GSH into GSSG; NADPH helps to regenerate GSH, thus preventing oxidative stress in the RBCs

- Since the hemoglobin and erythrocyte membrane are protected from damage by reduced glutathione (GSH), deficiency of the enzyme G6PD and in turn NADPH and in turn GSH produce two major events:
    - erythrocyte membrane damage
    - oxidation and denaturation of hemoglobin (forming Heinz bodies)

- **Epidemiology**
- G6PD deficiency is the most common metabolic disorder of erythrocytes and the most common human enzyme defect
- More than 400 million people worldwide are affected
- Though global in distribution, prevalence is greatest in malaria-endemic regions of the world, including West Africa, the Mediterranean, Middle East and South-East Asia

- **Mode of inheritance**
- G6PD deficiency is inherited as an X-linked recessive disorder
- The gene coding for the enzyme is located on the X-chromosome (band Xq 28)
- Male and homozygous females are affected; while heterozygous females are carriers
- Rarely, heterozygous female can be affected; this is may be due to inactivation of the normal X-chromosome (lyonization hypothesis)

- **Clinical Features**
- There are four main syndromes associated with G6PD deficiency; they are:
  - Acute hemolysis
  - Favism
  - Congenital nonspherocytic hemolytic anemia (CNSHA)
  - Drug-induced hemolytic anaemia

- **Acute hemolysis**
- This is the sudden destruction of enzyme-deficient erythrocytes.
- It is usually triggered by drugs, infectious agents or metabolic disorders e.g diabetic keto acidosis
- Hemolysis is usually intravascular

- **Favism**
  - This is an acute hemolytic anemia caused by ingestion of fava beans or inhalation of the pollen of the plant *Vicia faba* (Fava) in an individual with G6PD
  - Favism occurs most commonly in children between ages 1 - 5 years

- **Congenital nonspherocytic hemolytic anemia (CNSHA)**
  - This occurs in only a small fraction of G6PD-deficient individuals.
  - They develop a chronic life-long hemolysis in the absence of trigger factors
  - Beyond infancy, features of the disorder are subtle and inconstant.
  - Pallor is observed infrequently, jaundice is noted intermittently, and rarely the spleen is enlarged

- **Drug-induced haemolytic anaemia**
  - Drugs having a high redox potential are known to induce hemolysis in G6PD deficient patient
  - The common denominator of these drugs is that they interact with hemoglobin and oxygen, thus accelerating the intracellular formation of hydrogen peroxide (H_2O_2) and other oxidizing radicals.
  - The following are examples of drugs that may trigger acute hemolysis:

• Primaquine	• β-naphthol
• Procainamide	• Sulfamethoxypyridazine
• Pyrimethamine	• Sulfisoxazole
• Quinidine	• Trimethoprim
• Quinine	• Vitamin K
• Streptomycin	• Co-trimoxazole
• Fansidar	

- **Neonatal jaundice**
- G6PD deficiency is one of the commonest cause of neonatal jaundice in this environment
- It is usually prolonged and may lead to kernicterus

- **Others features**
- Dark brown urine (hemoglobinuria)
- Splenomegaly
- Fatigue
- Pallor
- Tachycardia
- Shortness of breath
- Acute renal failure (in severe hemolytic anemia)

- **Laboratory diagnosis**
- **Screening Tests**
- Several screening tests have been devised to identify G6PDdeficiency in red blood cells. The most widely used ones are:
- the Brilliant Cresyl blue decolorization test
- the Methemoglobin reduction test and
- an Ultraviolet spot test

- These tests can reliably distinguish between deficient or not deficient individuals, but are not reliably quantitative.

- Hemizygous   deficient   males   and   homozygous   deficient   females will be identified, the threshold being a G6PD activity of about 30% of normal.

- **Spectrophotometric assay**
- If the screening test indicates deficiency or is doubtful, this test is the ideal follow-up test for diagnostic quantification of the enzyme activity

- **DNA analysis: for definitive diagnosis**

- **Other supportive tests**
- Bilirubin level (increase)
- Full blood count (decrease)
- Hemoglobin level in the blood (increase)
- Hemoglobin level in the urine (increase)
- Haptoglobin level (decrease)
- Reticulocyte count (increase)
- Lactate dehydrogenase level (increase)
- Direct antiglobulin test (negative)

- **Treatment**
- Management of the patient with G6PD deficiency is determined by the clinical syndrome with which the patient present:
- Stop the offending drug or food
- Treat any underlying infection
- Maintain a high urine output by ensuring adequate rehydration
- Blood transfusion; in severe anemia
- Phototherapy or exchange blood transfusion in neonatal jaundice; to prevent kernicterus

- Dialysis in acute renal failure
- Vitamin E supplement; due to its antioxidant properties
- Vaccination against infectious agents

✓ Splenectomy is generally not beneficial

❖ **PYRUVATE KINASE (PK) DEFICIENCY**

▪ **Introduction**
- Pyruvate kinase (PK) deficiency is an inherited metabolic disorder, characterised by an abnormally low level of the enzyme pyruvate kinase in the red cell, causing chronic hemolytic anemia of widely variable severity
- It is the most common glycolytic enzyme defect in the Embden-Meyerhof pathway

▪ **Normal function of PK and Pathophysiology of PK deficiency**
- Pyruvate kinase is the enzyme which catalyses the final step of the glycolytic pathway where phosphoenolpyruvate (PEP) is converted to pyruvate, along with substrate level phosphorylation of ADP to ATP
- Thus, in PK deficiency, pyruvate cannot be produced and in turn ATP cannot be generated; causing lack of energy required for normal erythrocyte functions
- The cells become rigid and fragile, making them susceptible to hemolysis

▪ **Epidemiology**
- Most cases of PK deficiency have been reported from Northern Europe, the United States, and Japan; however, the disorder occurs worldwide.

- A prevalence of PK deficiency has been estimated to be 51 per million population.

- **Mode of inheritance**
- PK deficiency is inherited as an autosomal recessive disorder
- Thus, homozygous or doubly heterozygous individual are affected

- **Molecular biology**
- Four isoenzymes of pyruvate kinase exit in different tissues.
- The four isoenzymes are derived from two separate genes; two from each gene
- The *PKM* gene, on chromosome 15, produces PKM1 and PKM2.

  - PKM1 is found in skeletal muscles
  - PKM2 in leucocytes, kidneys, adipose tissue and lungs.

- The second PK gene (PKLR), on chromosome 1, gives rise to PKL and PKR
  - PKL is present in the liver
  - PKR is present in red cells.

- However, PK deficiency occurs due to mutation of the PKLR gene (1q21) which causes deficiency in the liver and erythrocyte isoenzyme of PK.

- **Clinical features**
- Hemolytic anemia in the newborn
- Pronounced neonatal jaundice
- Failure to thrive
- Aplastic crisis (caused by parvovirus B19)
- Gall stones (usually after the first decade of life)

- Frontal bossing (due to bone marrow hyperplasia)
- Right hypochondriac tenderness
- Splenomegaly (mild to moderate)
- Chronic leg ulcer (rarely)

- **Laboratory diagnosis**
- **Full blood count**
- Anemia (Hb conc of 6 - 12 g/dl)

- **Peripheral blood smear**
- Shows normochromic anemia with reticulocytosis, polychromatophilia, anisocytosis, poikilocytosis and variable number of nucleated erythrocytes

- **Direct DNA analysis**
- Useful for prenatal diagnosis

- **Other tests**
- Specific enzyme screening tests
- Bilirubin level
- Haptoglobin level
- Stool urobilinogen

- **Treatment**
- **Red cell transfusion: for treating severe anemia in the first year of life**
- **Splenectomy**
- Useful for long-term control of anemia
- However, surgery should be delayed till after 5 yrs to minimize the risk of post-splenectomy sepsis due to *Streptococcus pneumoniae*

- **Bone marrow transplantation**
- The risk-benefit ratio is currently in favour of splenectomy

CHAPTER 11: ANEMIA DUE TO NUTRIENT DEFICIENCY

❖ IRON DEFICIENCY ANEMIA (IDA)

- **Introduction**
- Though, iron is the fourth most common element in the earth's crust, its deficiency is the most common cause of anemia in every countries of the world!
- It affects about 500 million people world wide

- **Dietary source of iron**

Sources of heme iron	Sources of Inorganic iron
Meat (especially liver)	Beans
Shrimp	Almond
Oyster	Bread
Salmon	Rice

- **Absorption of iron**
- Dietary iron is absorbed from the duodenum and jejunum in Fe^{2+} form
- Heme Fe is better absorbed; however, most dietary iron is in the inorganic form
- Only 5-10% of the total iron in diet is usually absorbed
- However, in pregnancy and iron deficient state, absorption is increased to about 30%
- Some factors favour and others reduce the rate of iron absorption

Factors reducing iron absorption	Factors favouring iron absorption
Ferric form (Fe^{3+})	Ferrous form (Fe^{2+})
Antacids	Reducing sugar
Phytates	Vitamin C
Calcium	Iron deficiency

Tannins in tea	Hydrochloric acid
Infection	Pregnancy
Pancreatic secretion	Heme
Inorganic ions	
Alkali	
Increased Hepcidin	
Iron excess	

- **Body iron distribution and transport**
- The transport and storage of iron is largely mediated by 3 proteins: transferring, transferrin receptor 1 (TfR1), ferritin

- **Transferrin**
- Iron is transported in plasma bound to transferrin (an 80,000 molecular weight protein produced by the liver)
- Each molecule binds two atoms of ferric iron (Fe^{3+}) and delivers them to tissues having the transferrin receptor (TfR1) especially erythroblasts of the bone marrow for re-utilization
- The irons on transferrin are those released from destroyed RBCs in the reticuloendothelial system and only a small portion is of dietary origin
- Note that, when iron level is low, plasma transferrin level rises, and when iron level is high, plasma transferrin falls

- **Ferritin and Hemosiderin**
- Ferritin and hemosiderin are storage forms of iron in the macrophage

- **Ferritin**
- It is a water soluble complex of iron and protein, having a molecular weight of 465,000
- Each molecule binds up to 4000 - 5000 atoms of iron
- It is not visible under light microscope

- **Hemosiderin**
  - It is a water insoluble complex of iron (in ferric form) and protein
  - It binds more iron molecule than ferritin
  - It is formed by partial digestion of aggregates of ferritin molecules
  - It is visible in macrophages and other cells via light microscopy following staining by Perl's reaction (Prussian blue)
  - Iron can only be mobilized from it, after its reduction to Fe^{2+}; a vitamin C-dependent reaction

- **Hepcidin**
  - Hepcidin is a 25 amino acid polypeptide produced by the liver
  - It is a major regulator of iron homeostasis and as well an acute phase protein
  - It inhibits Fe release from macrophages, intestinal epithelial cells and placental syncytiotrophoblasts
  - Its secretion is inhibited in iron deficiency, hypoxia and ineffective erythropoiesis

- **Causes of iron deficiency anemia**
- **Gastrointestinal**
  - Hook worm infestation
  - Bleeding esophageal varices
  - Partial gatrectomy
  - Gluten-induced enteropathy
  - Achlorhydria
  - Chronic atrophic gastritis

- **Increased demand**
  - Prematurity
  - Lactation
  - Pregnancy

- Menstruation
- Growth
- Erythropoietin therapy

- **Poor diet**
- Only contributory (rarely the sole cause)

- In developing countries; hookworm infestation leading to chronic blood loss, is the commonest cause of iron deficiency
- In developed countries; non-parasitic gastrointestinal blood loss in adult males and menstrual blood loss in perimenopausal females are the common causes.

- **Progression of iron deficiency**
- All storage forms of iron (ferritin and hemosiderin) must have been completely depleted before IDA appears
- Iron deficiency follows a typical pattern of progression; as shown below:

- **Clinical features of IDA**
- **General features of anemia**
- Weakness / undue tiredness
- Easy fatigability
- Lethargy
- Palpitation
- Headache
- Pallor
- Tachycardia
- Bounding pulse
- Cardiomegaly
- Systemic flow murmur

- **Specific features of IDA**

- Painless glossitis (glossy tongue with atrophy of lingual papillae)
- Angular stomatitis (fissures and ulcers at the corners of the mouth)
- Spoon–shaped nails (koilonychia)
- Unusual dietary cravings (Pica)
- Dysphagia with solid foods, due to post-cricoid esophageal webbing (Plummer-Vinson or Paterson-Brown Kelly syndrome)
- Leg cramping (on climbing stairs)
- Poor cognitive function
- Decline in psychomotor development
- Irritability
- Cold intolerance

- **Diagnosis and laboratory findings in IDA**
- **Peripheral blood smear**
- Hypochromic microcytic anemia
- Target cells and pencil-shaped poikilocytes

- **Full blood count**
- Reduction in erythrocyte and platelet count
- Normal or mildly elevated leukocyte count

- **Red cell indices**
- Low MCV
- Low MCHC

- **Serum iron and total iron-binding capacity**
- Low serum iron and ferritin
- Increased total iron binding capacity

- Bone marrow iron
- Complete absence of iron from marrow stores (macrophages) and erythroblasts
- Increased level of serum transferrin receptor (sTfR)

- Treatment
- Investigate the cause and treat accordingly
- Give iron supplement (to correct the anemia and replenish iron stores)

- Forms of iron preparations
- ✓ Oral iron
- Ferrous sulphate
- This is best oral iron preparation
- Given daily (200mg) on empty stomach 6hrly for about 6 months
- The Hb should rise at the rate of 2g/dL every 3wks
- Note that the elemental iron in one tablet of ferrous sulphate(200mg) is only 67mg

- Ferrous gluconate
- The elemental iron in one tablet of ferrous gluconate(300mg) is only 37mg

- Side Effect of oral iron
- Nausea
- Abdominal pain
- Constipation
- Diarrhoea

- ✓ Parenteral iron

- This is reserved only for patient who cannot absorb or tolerate oral iron
- They include:

- **Ferric hydroxide sucrose (venofer)**
- The safest parenteral preparation
- Given slowly intravenously

- **Iron sorbitol citrate (Jectofer)**
- Given intramuscularly

- **Iron dextran**
- Available as intramuscular and intravenous preparations

- **Side Effect**
- Anaphylactic reaction
- Athralgia
- Fever
- Hypotension

- ❖ MEGALOBLASTIC ANEMIA

- **Introduction**
- Megaloblastic anemia is a group of anemias characterised by presence of megaloblasts in the bone marrow
- Megaloblasts are large, nucleated, immature progenitor of an abnormal red blood cell series that correspond to the erythroblasts of normal erythropoiesis
- They show delayed maturation of nucleus relative to the cytoplasm
- The underlying defect accounting for the asynchronous maturation of erythroblasts is defective DNA synthesis; which manifests as delayed nuclear maturation

- Causes of MA
- In clinical practise, the most common causes of megaloblastic anemia are:
  - Vitamin B_{12} deficiency
  - Folate deficiency

- Less common causes
- These are mainly abnormalities in the metabolism of folic acid and vitamin B_{12}, or other lesions in DNA synthesis; they include:
  - Transcobalamin deficiency
  - Nitrous oxide
  - Anti-folate drugs (methotrexate, pyrimethamine trimethoprim etc.)
  - Orotic aciduria
  - Alcohol

- Physiology of vitamin B_{12}
- **Food source**
- Vitamin B_{12} is found only in food of animal origin; examples are: meat (especially liver), fish, diary products

- **Absorption**
- It is absorbed by combining with intrinsic factors (secreted by gastric parietal cells) to form IF-B_{12} complex
- The complex in turn binds to other proteins (cubilin and amionless) which assist in its final absorption in the distal ileum

- **Transport**
- Vitamin B_{12} now in the portal blood attaches to transcobalamin (its plasma binding protein) which delivers it to the bone marrow and other tissue for utilization.

- **Metabolism**
- Vitamin B_{12} acts as co-enzyme for two biochemical reactions in the body:

- In form of methylcobalamine, vitamin B_{12} act as coenzyme for the enzyme methionine synthase; involved in methylation of homocysteine to methionine
- In form of deoxyadenosyl cobalamin, vitamin B_{12} assists in the conversion of methyl malonyl CoA to succinyl CoA

- **Physiology of Folic acid**
- **Food source**
- Folate is derive from food of both animal and plant origin; examples are: liver, yeast, spinach, nuts, green vegetable

- **Absorption**
- Folate is absorbed from the upper small intestine, during which it is converted to methyl tetrahydrofolate; the form in which all body cells receive it
- Once inside the cell, they are converted to folate polyglutamates
- Total body folate is 10mg, and the daily requirement is 100ug

- **Metabolism**
- Folate is required in a variety of biochemical reactions in the body:
- Amino acid interconvertion e.g. conversion of homocysteine to methionine and serine to glycine
- Synthesis of purine precursors of DNA (i.e. adenine and guanine)

- Biochemical basis of megaloblastic anemia
- The etiology of megaloblastic anemia is impaired DNA synthesis and assembly; resulting most commonly from folate and/or vitamin B_{12} deficiency
- Folate deficiency impair the synthesis of thymidylate (a precursor of thymine)
- Since thymine is a DNA building block, a limitation in its supply will impair DNA synthesis; leading to delay in nuclear maturation
- Vitamin B_{12} deficiency impair the conversion of methyl tetrahydrofolate to tetrahydrofolate (THF); a reaction essential for the formation of methionine from homocysteine
- Tetrahydrofolate (THF) is the substrate for synthesis of folate polyglutamates inside the cell
- The folate polyglutamates act as intracellular folate coenzyme involved in thymidylate synthetase reaction for thymidylate synthesis
- Thus, impairment of THF formation due to Vitamin B_{12} deficiency causes delay in DNA synthesis and delayed nuclear maturation

- Causes of Vitamin B_{12} deficiency
- Nutritional: especially in vegans
- Malabsorption
- Pernicious anemia
- Congenital lack or abnormality of intrinsic factor
- Total or partial gastrectomy
- Intestinal stagnant loop syndrome
- Chronic tropical sprue
- Ileal resection and Crohn's disease

Causes of Vitamin B_{12} deficiency

- **Nutritional:** old age, poverty, goat milk

- **Malabsorption: tropical sprue, gluten-induced enteropathy, partial gastrectomy**
- **Excessive utilization: pregnancy, lactation, malignancy**
- **Drugs:** anticonvulsant, sulfasalazine, alcohol

Clinical features of MA

- **General features of anemia**
- **Specific features of MA**
- Painful glossitis
- Angular stomatitis
- Weight loss
- Purpura (due to thrombocytopenia)
- Widespread melanin pigmentation
- Increased incidence of infection
- Premature grey hair and blue eye
- Peripheral neuropathy (for B_{12} only)
- Sterility (affects either sex)
- Decreased osteoblast activity
- Neural tube defect in the fetus

- **Laboratory Findings in MA**
- **Full blood count**
- Reticulocyte count is low
- Total leukocyte and platelet count may be moderately reduced

- **Peripheral blood smear**
- Presence of macrocytes
- Neutrophils show hypersegmented nuclei (6 or more lobes)

- **Bone marrow examination**
- Bone marrow is hypercellular (filled with megaloblasts)

— Presence of giant and abnormally shaped metamyelocyte

- **Biochemical tests**
— Serum and red cell folate level (decreased)
— Serum vitamin B_{12} level (decreased)
— Serum bilirubin (increased)
— Serum lactate dehydrogenase (LDH) level (increased)

- Treatment
— Most cases of megaloblastic anemia only need treatment with the appropriate vitamin

	Vitamin B12 deficiency	Folic acid deficiency
Compound	Hydroxocobalamin	Folic acid
Route of administration	Intramuscular	Oral
Dose	1000 µg	5mg
Initial dose	6 x 1000 µg over 2-3wks	Daily for 4month
Maintenance	1000 µg every 3 months	Depends on underlying disease; life-long therapy may be needed in chronic inherited hemolytic anemias, myelofibrosis, renal dialysis

CHAPTER 12: ACQUIRED HEMOLYTIC ANEMIAS

- Acquired hemolytic anemia are hemolytic anemia resulting from non-hereditary causes or defect extrinsic to the red blood cells
- Broadly, they are divided into two:

- Immune hemolytic anemia
- Non-Immune hemolytic anemia

❖ IMMUNE HEMOLYTIC ANEMIAS (IHA)

■ **Introduction**

- Immune hemolytic anemia occurs when antibodies are formed against red cells following exposure to drugs, toxins or other antigens, resulting in their massive destruction and consequently anemia

■ **Antibody**

- Antibodies are immunoglobulin molecules produced by B lymphoid cells following exposure to an antigen

● **Types of antibody**

✓ **Autoantibody**

- These are antibodies formed in response to and reacting against, a self antigen i.e. one of the individual's own normal tissue constituent (in this case the erythrocytes)

✓ **Alloantibody (isoantibody)**

- These are antibodies formed in response to and reacting against, the antigen of another individual of the same species

- Classification of antibody
- Cold antibody
  - They are usually IgM, but occasionally IgG
  - They display increasing activity against red cells as temperature approaches 0^0C
  - They fix compliments and may lead to immediate intravascular red cell destruction or their removal from the circulation by the liver

- **Warm antibody**
  - These are typically IgG
  - They display increasing activity against red cells as temperature approaches 37^0C
  - They may or may not fix compliment
  - They primarily lead to destruction of sensitized RBCs by the spleen

- Classification of IHA
  - Immune hemolytic anemias are broadly classified into two:

- Autoimmune hemolytic anemia
- Alloimmune hemolytic anemia

❖ AUTOIMMUNE HEMOLYTIC ANEMIAS (AIHAs)
  - Autoimmune hemolytic anemias (AHIAs) are a group of anemias characterized by production of autoantibodies, by the body, against its own red cells

- Classification of AIHAs
  - According to whether the autoantibody reacts more strongly with red cells at 37°C or 0°C AIHAs can be classified as:
    - Warm antibody type AIHA
    - Cold antibody type AIHA

- **Warm antibody type AIHA**
- **Pathophysiology**
  - The RBCs are coated with immunoglobulin G (IgG) with or without complement proteins
  - The sensitized RBCs are in turn taken up by reticulo-endothelial macrophages through their receptor for Fc fragment of the immunoglobulin
  - The cells progressively lose the coated part of their membrane and become more spherical; though their volume remain the same
  - Ultimately they are prematurely destroyed, predominantly in the spleen.

- **Classification**
  - Warm antibody type AIHA can be sub-classified based on the etiology as:
    - Primary/idiopathic
    - Secondary

- **Primary/idiopathic warm antibody type AIHA**
  - Here, no disorder is found responsible for the AIHA
  - It is commoner in female and children

- **Clinical feature**
  - Symptoms of anemia
  - Pallor
  - Jaundice
  - Splenomegaly (mild to moderate)
  - Evan's syndrome

❖ Evan's syndrome

- This is the association of idiopathic warm antibody type AIHA with immune thrombocytopenia

▪ Secondary warm antibody type AIHA

- Here, the AIHA is attributable to particular etiology
- Table 12.1 summarizes the various disorders that may precipitate secondary warm antibody type AIHA

Disorder	Examples
Autoimmune disease	Systemic lupus erythematosus (SLE) Rheumatoid arthritis Sjogren's syndrome Ulcerative colitis
Lymphoproliferative disorders	B-cell chronic lymphocytic leukemia (CLL) Low grade B-cell non-Hodgkin's lymphoma Hodgkin's Lymphoma
Drugs	Penicillin, Methyldopa, Quinidine, L-dopa Mefenamic acid, Procainamide etc
Carcinomas	Ovarian cyst, Ovarian carcinoma
Viral infections	
Immune deficiency states	

▪ Laboratory Diagnosis of warm antibody types AIHA

● **Direct antiglobulin test**

- This test detects antibodies or compliments bound to red cell surface in vivo
- The antihuman globulin (AHG) reagent is added to washed red cells
- Agglutination indicates a positive test
- It is positive in warm AIHA (and in hemolytic transfusion reaction)

- **Peripheral blood smear**
- Evidence of extravascular hemolysis and prominent spherocytosis are seen in the peripheral blood

- **Treatment warm antibody types AIHA**
- Remove the underlying cause
- Corticosteroid (usually prednisolone)
- Splenectomy (if patient is not responding to other lines of management)
- Immunosuppression; using azathriopine, cyclophosphamide etc. (when other measures have failed)
- Monoclonal antibodies e.g. rituximab (anti-CD20) or alemtuzumab a.k.a. Campath-1H (anti-CD 52)

- **Cold antibody type AIHA**
- **Pathophysiology**
- The RBCs are coated with immunoglobulin M (IgM) which binds red cells best at 4°C
- The binding occurs mainly in the peripheral circulation; where temperature is cool.
- Following binding, IgM fix compliment proteins which results in both intravascular and extravascular hemolysis

- **Classification**
- Cold antibody type AIHA can be sub-classified based on the etiology as:

- Cold hemagglutinin disease
- Cold agglutinin syndrome

- **Cold hemagglutinin disease**
- This is mostly seen in older people and runs a chronic course

- Etiology is unknown

- **Cold agglutinin disease**
- Here, etiology of the hemolysis is known
- It may follow the following disorders:

- **Lymphoproliferative disease:** B-cell lymphoma, CLL

- Infection: Mycoplasma pneumonia, infectious mononucleosis, Listeriosis, Toxoplasmosis

- Clinical features of cold antibody type AIHA
- **Chronic hemolytic anemia:** aggravated by cold; hemolysis is commonly intravascular
- **Acrocyanosis:** bluish discolouration of the tip of the nose, ears, and digits
- Mild jaundice
- Splenomegaly

- Laboratory Diagnosis of warm antibody types AIHA
- **Direct antiglobulin test: as described above, It is positive in cold AIHA**
- **Peripheral blood smear: spherocytosis is less marked**

- Treatment
- Keep the patient warm
- Treat underlying etiology
- Alkylating agent e.g. chlorambucil may be helpful in chronic varieties
- Monoclonal antibodies e.g. rituximab (anti-CD20) or alemtuzumab a.k.a. Campath-1H (anti-CD 52) have been used

✓ Splenectomy is not helpful here, as hemolysis is usually intravascular; except of course if the enlargement is massive
✓ Steroids are not helpful here

❖ **ALLOIMMUNE HEMOLYTIC ANEMIA**
− In this type of immune hemolytic anemia, antibodies (alloantibodies a.k.a. isoantibodies) produced by an individual reacts against the RBCs from another individual
− The two important examples of this are:
  • ABO incompatibility
  • Rhesus isoimmunisation

SECTION III   HEMOSTASIS

CHAPTER 13: INTRODUCTION TO HEMOSTASIS

■ **Definition**

— Hemostasis is the process of arrest of bleeding from an injured blood vessel, without interrupting blood flow through it

— It requires the contribution of various component of the hemostatic system:
  • Vascular endothelium
  • Platelets
  • Plasma proteins (mainly by the liver)

■ **Coagulation factors**

— These are substances in the blood that are essential to the clotting process and hence to the maintenance of normal hemostasis.

— All except factors III and IV are synthesised by the liver; they include:

- Factor I – Fibrinogen
- Factor II – prothrombin
- Factor III* – tissue factor/thromboplastin
- Factor IV* – calcium ions
- Factor V – labile factor
- Factor VII – stable factor
- Factor VIII – antihemophilic factor
- Factor IX – Christmas factor
- Factor X – Stuart-Prower factor
- Factor XI – plasma thromboplastin antecedent
- Factor XII – Hageman factor
- Factor XIII – Fibrin stabilizing factor

❖ **Mechanism of hemostasis**

– Arrest of bleeding from an injured blood vessel occurs in the following sequence:
  • Vasoconstriction
  • Platelet plug formation
  • Blood coagulation
  • Clot formation and retraction
  • Fibrinolysis

■ **Vasoconstriction**

– This is the narrowing (large vessels) or occlusion (small vessels) of the lumen of the injured blood vessel, so as to reduce or stop blood loss
– Mediators include; endothelin, thromboxane A_2, direct stimulation of the vessel wall by the injurious agent, and nervous reflexes initiated by pain impulses

■ **Platelet plug formation / primary hemostasis**

– Damage to the vascular endothelial lining causes exposure of collagen from the basement membrane
– Free flowing platelets contacts and adhere to the collagen; mediated by vWF
– The adhered platelets degranulate and release ADP; which initiate prostaglandin synthesis (especially TXA_2)
– The released ADP and TXA_2 attract and activate other free flowing platelets to adhere to the injured site
– Eventually an aggregate of platelets called platelet plug fill the site

■ **Blood coagulation / secondary hemostasis**

– This is the sequential process by which the multiple coagulation factors in blood interact in the coagulation cascade to ultimately produce an insoluble fibrin clot

- Blood coagulation occurs in three stages:
  - Formation of prothrombin activator
  - Conversion of prothrombin to thrombin
  - Conversion of fibrinogen into fibrin

- Formation of prothrombin activator
  - Prothrombin activator, which helps in the conversion prothrombin to thrombin, can be formed in any of two pathways:

✓ Extrinsic pathway
- Tissue factor (FIII) is released from the damaged endothelium;
- The glycoprotein and phospholipid component of tissue factor (FIII) converts factor X (FX) into activated factor X (FXa) in the presence of factor VII
- FXa reacts with factor V and phospholipid component of tissue factor (FIII) in the presence of calcium ion to form prothrombin activator.

✓ Intrinsic pathway
- Following injury, the blood vessel is ruptured, endothelium is damaged and collagen is exposed.
- When factor XII (FXII) comes in contact with collagen, it is converted into activated factor XII (FXIIa) in the presence of kallikrein and kinogen.
- FXIIa converts factor XI into activated factor XI (FXIa) in the presence of kinogen.
- FXIa activates factor IX in the presence of factor IV (calcium).
- FIXa activates factor X in the presence of factor VIII and calcium.
- When platelet comes in contact with collagen of damaged blood vessel, it gets activated and releases phospholipids.

- Now FXa reacts with platelet phos pholipid and factor V to form prothrombin activator

- **Conversion of prothrombin to thrombin**
- Prothrombin activator formed in intrinsic and extrinsic pathways converts prothrombin into thrombin in the presence of calcium

- **Conversion of fibrinogen into fibrin**
- The final stage of blood clotting involves the conversion of fibrinogen into fibrin by thrombin

- **Clot retraction**
- It occurs after clot formation
- It requires a large number of platelets
- It contributes to hemostasis by squeezing serum from the clot and joining the edges of the broken vessel

- **Fibrinolysis**
- This is the dissolution of fibrin; to remove excess clot from lumen of the blood vessel
- It requires an enzyme called plasmin or fibrinolysin

CHAPTER 14: BLEEDING DISORDERS

- Introduction
- Bleeding disorders a.k.a. clotting disorder or coagulopathy, is a condition characterized by impaired ability of blood to clot; causing prolonged and excessive bleeding

- Classification of bleeding disorders
- Impairment of coagulation can result from disorders affecting any of the factors contributing to hemostasis; thus they are divided into 3 main groups:
- Vascular disorders
- Platelet disorders
- Coagulation disorders

- Definition of terms
- **Petechiae:** pinpoint cutaneous hemorrhages about 1-2mm in diameter
- **Purpura:** cutaneous hemorrhages > 3mm but < 1cm in diameter
- **Ecchymosis:** cutaneous hemorrhages > 1 cm in diameter

❖ VASCULAR DISORDERS

- Introduction
- Here, the underlying abnormality is either in the vessels themselves or in the perivascular connective tissues

- Characteristics of vascular disorders
- Most cases are usually not severe i.e. blood loss is not serious
- Bleeding is mainly into the skin; causing petechiae, purpura or both

- The various tests of hemostasis are normal; including the bleeding time
- May be inherited of acquired

- **Inherited vascular disorders: These include:**
- **Hereditary haemorrhagic telangiectasia**
- **Connective tissue disorders:**
  - . Ehlers-Danlos syndrome
  - . Pseudoxanthoma elasticum
  - . Marfan syndrome
  - − Giant cavernous hemangioma

- **Hereditary haemorrhagic telangiectasia**
- An autosomal dominant disorder
- Dilated and swollen microvasculatures appear in childhood and increases with age
- Telangiectasia (permanent dilatation of pre-existing blood vessels) develop in the skin, mucous membrane and internal organ

- **Ehlers-Danlos syndrome**
- An hereditary fibrillar collagen deficiency, causing defective platelet aggregation

- **Giant cavernous hemangioma**
- A congenital malformation which occasionally causes chronic activation of the coagulation cascade
- It causes thrombocytopenia in some cases

- **Acquired vascular disorders: these include:**
- Scurvy

- Senile purpura
- Steroid purpura
- Infection
- Henoch-Schonlein syndrome purpura
- Psychogenic purpura (Gardner-diamond syndrome)

- **Scurvy**
- A manifestation of vitamin C deficiency;
- Associated with production of weak collagen strands, which predisposes to capillary fragility and impaired wound healing

- **Senile purpura**
- Caused by atrophy of vascular supporting tissue due to old age

- **Steroid purpura**
- Caused by defect in vascular supporting tissue due to prolonged steroid therapy or Cushing syndrome

- **Treatment: Treat the underlying cause**

CHAPTER 15: PLATELET DISORDERS

- **Introduction**
- Here, the underlying abnormality responsible for the bleeding is either a deficiency in the number of platelet (quantitative) or a defect in their function (qualitative)

- **Characteristics Platelet disorders**
- Bleeding is mainly into the skin and mucosa ; causing petechiae, purpura or both
- Bleeding time is prolonged
- Sex distribution is equal
- May be inherited of acquired

- **Classification of Platelet disorders**
- Thrombocytopenias (deficiency in number)
- Thrombocytopathies (defect in function)

- ❖ THROMBOCYTOPENIAS
- By definition; thrombocytopenia is a lower than normal number of platelets in the blood; usually when below 50,000/µL
- Though platelet count is low, their function usually remain completely intact

- **Subdivisions of thrombocytopenia**
- Congenital thrombocytopenias (inherited or non-inherited)
- Acquired thrombocytopenias

- ■ Congenital Thrombocytopenias
- ● **Inherited congenital Thrombocytopenias**

Inherited congenital thrombocytopenias	Inheritance /Defect	Clinical features
Wiskott-Aldrich syndrome (WAS)	X-linked recessive	Eczema, Thrombocytopenia, Recurrent infections
X-linked thrombocytopenia (XLT)	X-linked recessive	Thrombocytopenia +/- Features of WAS
Congenital amegakaryocytic thrombocytopenia (CAMT)	Autosomal recessive	Bone marrow aplasia, Abnormalities of thrombopoietin (c-mpl) receptor
Thrombocytopenia with absent radii (TAR)	Autosomal recessive	Feature of CAMT bilateral agenesis of radius Severe hemorrhage
Shulman-Upshaw syndrome	ADAM TS13 mutation	Thrombotic thrombocytopenic purpura (TTP) Thrombocytopenia
May-Hegglin anomaly	Autosomal dominant	Giant platelet Thrombocytopenia Dohle bodies in granulocytes
Grey platelet syndrome (GPS)	Autosomal dominant	Large platelet Thrombocytopenia

- ■ **Non-inherited congenital thrombocytopenias**
- – These are thrombocytopenias resulting from agents or disorders which induce deficient platelet production or enhanced platelet destruction
- – It may be due to any of the following situation:
  - • Maternal use of drugs and chemical agents
  - • Isoimmune thrombocytopenia
  - • Infiltration of bone marrow
  - • Infection

- **Acquired Thrombocytopenias**
- These account by far for most cases of thrombocytopenia; and may be due to any of the following mechanisms:
    - Failure of platelet production
    - Increased destruction of platelets
    - Abnormal distribution of platelets (due to splenomegaly)
    - Dilutional loss (due to massive blood transfusion)

❖ **THROMBOCYTOPATHIES**
- By definition; thrombocytopathy is any disorder of coagulation resulting from platelet dysfunction
- Thus, bleeding is not arrested even in the presence of normal platelet count

- **Subdivisions of thrombocytopathies**
- Inherited thrombocytopathies
- Acquired thrombocytopathies

- **Inherited Thrombocytopathies**
- These are usually rare disorders
- The defect may be at any of the phases of platelet reactions
- Examples are:
    - Glanzmann's thrombasthenia
    - Bernard-Soulier syndrome
    - Storage pool deficiency syndromes:
        - Grey platelet syndrome
        - β-storage pool disease

- **Glanzmann's thrombasthenia**
- An autosomal recessive disorder

- Primary defect is deficiency of membrane glycoproteins IIb-IIIa complex
- Characterised by failure of platelet aggregation

• **Bernard-Soulier syndrome**
- An autosomal recessive disorder
- Primary defect is deficiency of membrane glycoproteins Ib
- Characterised by defective binding of platelet to vWF and in turn defective adherence to subendothelial connective tissue; and thus failure of platelet aggregation

• **Storage pool deficiency syndromes**
- These are the most common disorder of secondary platelet aggregation
- They include:

✓ **Grey platelet syndrome:** larger than normal platelet, and Virtual absence of α-granules
✓ **β-storage pool disease:** deficiency of dense granules

• **Acquired Thrombocytopathies**
- These are more common causes of thrombocytopathy
- Causes include:
  • Antiplatelet drugs
  • Hyperglobulinemia (e.g. in multiple myeloma, waldestrom's macroglobulinemia)
  • Myeloproliferative or myelodysplastic disorders
  • Uremia

• **Antiplatelet drugs:** e.g. aspirin, dipyridamole, clopidogrel, abciximab etc.

• **Aspirin:** commonest cause of thrombocytopathy

- It inhibits the enzyme cyclo-oxygenase; thus impair with synthesis of TXA_2
- Produces abnormal bleeding time; though purpura may not be obvious
- Defect lasts 7-10 days after a single dose

- **Dipyridamole:** inhibits platelet aggregation by blocking reuptake of adenosine
- **Clopidogrel:** inhibits binding of ADP to its platelet receptor

- Treatment
- Steroids
- Intravenous immunoglobulins
- Platelet transfusion (see indication below)
- Splenectomy

- **Indications for platelet transfusion**
- When patient is bleeding or going for invasive procedures and alternative therapies (steroids and IV Immunoglobulin) are not available
- In patient going for liver biopsy or lumbar puncture with platelet count $< 50 \times 10^9/L$
- Prophylactically in patients with platelet cotmts of $< 5\text{-}10 \times 10^9/L$

CHAPTER 16: COAGULATION DISORDERS

- **Introduction**
- Coagulation disorders are genetic or acquired abnormalities of clotting factors that may result in various bleeding disorders
- Deficiency of all clotting factors, except of factor XII, causes bleeding

- **Comparison of coagulation and platelet disorders**

Features	Coagulation disorders	Platelet disorders
Onset of bleeding	Delayed	Spontaneous
Mucosal bleeding	Rare	Common
Petechiae	Rare	Characteristic
Deep hematomas	Characteristic	Rare
Ecchymoses	Large and solitary	Small and multiple
Hemarthrosis	Characteristic	Rare
Bleeding from superficial cuts	Minimal	Persistent and often profuse
Sex of patient	80-90% are male	Equal

-

- **Classification of coagulation disorders**
- Hereditary coagulation disorder
- Acquired coagulation disorder

- ❖ **HEREDITARY COAGULATION DISORDER**
- Hereditary deficiency of all coagulation factors have been described; however, most are rare

- The few common ones include:
  - Hemophilia A (factor VIII deficiency)
  - Hemophilia B (factor IX deficiency)
  - Von willebrand disease (vWD)
  - Hemophilia C (factor XI deficiency)

- **Hemophilia A (Factor VIII Deficiency)**
  - This is the most common of the hereditary clotting factor deficiencies
  - It accounts for about 85% of all hemophilias
  - Also known as Classical hemophilia

- **Etiology**
  - Deficiency of Factor VIII (antihemophilic factor)

- **Mode of inheritance**
  - It is inherited as an X-linked recessive disorder in about 70% of cases
  - The remaining 30% arise from de novo spontaneous mutation

- **Molecular genetics**
  - Factor VIII is coded for by the gene at the tip of long arm of X-chromosome (Xq2.6)
  - About 50% of the patients have missense, frame-shift mutation or deletions in the factor VIII gene
  - Being an X-linked disorder, most patients are male and homozygous females
  - Heterozygous females are carriers except in those whom the normal X-chromosomes were inactivated (through lyonization)
  - Also turner syndrome (45 XO) patient, bearing the mutation, will manifest the disease; as they have a single X-chromosome

- **Incidence: about 1 in 10,000 males is born with factor VIII deficiency**
- **Pathophysiology**
  - Factor VIII is synthesised mainly in the liver and circulates in plasma as a complex with von willebrand factor (its carrier molecule)

- Its deficiency in classical hemophiliacs drastically slows down the rate of generation of activated factor X (FXa) despite the presence of all other coagulation factors and platelets in normal amount

- **Grading**
- In hemophilia A, the severity of disease or degree of bleeding is clearly related to the extent of factor VII deficiency; thus it is graded as mild, moderate or severe (table 16.2)

Grade	% FVIII activity	Clinical manifestation
Mild	>10-30	Minor bleeding after significant trauma
Moderate	2-10	Bleeding after minor trauma
Severe	<2	Frequent spontaneous bleeding into joint and soft tissues

- **Clinical features**
- Easy bruising
- Recurrent painful hemarthrosis (especially in the weight bearing joint)
- Muscle hematoma
- Massive operative and post-traumatic bleed
- Spontaneous hematuria and gastrointestinal bleeding
- Oropharyngeal bleeding (though uncommon, is life threatening)
- Spontaneous intracerebral hemorrhage (though uncommon, is an important cause of death)

- **Infant**
- Profuse post-circumcision hemorrhage
- Cephalhematoma
- Joint and soft tissue bleed (when they start to be active)

- **Laboratory Findings**
- Activated partial thromboplastin time (APTT) – **prolonged**
- Factor VIII clotting assay – **<50 μ/dL**
- **The following tests are Normal:** Prothrombin time, Bleeding time, Platelet count

- **Treatment**
- **Factor VIII replacement therapy**
- Using recombinant factor VIII
- bleeding is usually controlled when FVIII level is raised to 30-50% of normal

- **Desmopressin (DDAVP)**
- Used in increasing factor VIII level in mild hemophiliacs
- Following its infusion, 2-4 fold rise in patient FVIII level within 30-60min
- Since it is a diuretic, it should be avoided in the elderly

- **Gene therapy has also been tried**

- **Hemophilia B (Factor IX Deficiency)**
- The second most common form of hemophilia
- Rarer than but clinically similar to hemophilia A
- Also known as Christmas disease

- **Etiology: deficiency of Factor IX (Christmas factor)**
- **Mode of inheritance: it is inherited as an X-linked recessive disorder**
- **Molecular genetics**
- Factor IX is coded for by a gene close to that for FVIII, near the tip of long arm of X-chromosome (Xq)

- Being an X-linked disorder, most patients are male and homozygous females
- Heterozygous females may manifest the disease (lyonization hypothesis)

- **Incidence: about 1 in 100,000 males is born with factor IX deficiency**
- **Grading**
- As in hemophilia A, severity of hemophilia B is clearly related to the extent of factor IX deficiency; thus it is also graded as mild, moderate or severe (as for hemophilia A)

- **Clinical features: as for hemophilia A**
- **Laboratory findings: as for hemophilia A**

- **Treatment**
- **Factor IX replacement therapy**
- Using high-purity factor IX or recombinant factor IX

- **Von Willebrand Disease (VWD)**
- von Willebrand disease (vWD) is an inheritable bleeding disorder characterised by a defect in von Willebrand factor (vWF)
- With an estimated frequency of 1%, vWD is believed to be the most common inherited bleeding disorder described in human

- **Von willebrand factor (vWF)**
- A glycoprotein synthesised in the endothelial cells and megakaryocytes that circulates in plasma complexed to FVIII; and has two main functions:
    - It serves as carrier molecule for FVIII; protecting it from premature destruction

- It mediates platelet adhesion to damaged endothelium

– Thus, occasionally, reduction in FVIII level is associated with vWD
– vWF is stored in weibel-palade bodies in endothelial cells as well as α-granules of platelets

- **Etiology**
– vWD occurs due either to a reduced level or abnormal function of vWF

- **Mode of inheritance**
– Mainly autosomal dominant (100) but may be rarely autosomal recessive (1)

- **Types of vWD**
– Three types of vWD exist; and are summarised in table....

Types	Description	Comment
1	Quantitative partial deficiency	Commonest type; account for 75% of vWD vWF function is normal but its synthesis is reduced
2	**Functional abnormality**	
2A	Decreased platelet function	Normal affinity of vWF for FVIII Absent HMW vWF multimers
2B	Increased affinity for GPIb	Normal affinity of vWF for FVIII reduced/absent HMW vWF multimers
2M	Decreased platelet function	Normal affinity of vWF for FVIII Normal or ultra large HMW vWF multimers
2N	Normal platelet function	Decreased affinity of vWF for FVIII Normal HMW vWF multimers
3	Complete deficiency	No detectable vWF activity Inheritance is autosomal recessive

GPIb – glycoprotein 1b, HMW - high molecular weight; vWF - von Willebrand factor

- **Clinical features**
- Mucous membrane bleeding (e.g. epistaxis, menorrhagia)
- Massive operative and post-traumatic bleed
- Hemarthroses and hematomas (only in type 3)

- **Laboratory findings**
- Bleeding time – prolonged
- FVIII level – low
- Activated partial thromboplastin time – prolonged
- vWF level – usually low
- Ristocetin-induced platelet aggregation is impaired
- Platelet count is normal except in type 2B disease

- **Treatment**
- **Antifibrinolytic agent**
- Example is epsilon-amino-caproic acid
- for mild bleeding

- **Desmopressin (DDAVP) infusion**
- For type 1 vWD;
- It releases vWF from endothelial stage sites 30 min after intravenous infusion

- **High-purity factor VWF concentrates**
- for patients with very low VWF levels

✓ *Factor VIII concentrate may also be given for more rapid correction.*

- **Hemophilia C (Factor XI Deficiency)**
- The least common of the hemophilias
- Caused by deficiency of factor XI

- Inheritance may be as autosomal dominant or recessive
- It affects both males and females
- Unlike in hemophilia A and B; risk of bleeding in hemophilia C is not always influenced by the severity of the deficiency

- **Other Clotting Factor Deficiency**
- They are rare
- All are inherited as autosomal recessive except dysfibrinogenemia which is inherited as autosomal dominant

❖ **ACQUIRED COAGULATION DISORDER**
- These are by far more common than the hereditary coagulation disorders
- Moreover, unlike in hereditary coagulation disorders where a single clotting factor is affected, multiple clotting factors are simultaneously affected in acquired coagulation disorders

- **Causes of acquired coagulation disorders**
- Vitamin K deficiency
- Liver disease
- Disseminated intravascular coagulation (DIC)
- Massive transfusion
- Drugs (e.g. antibiotics, anticancer etc.)

SECTION IV   BLOOD TRANSFUSION

CHAPTER 17: BLOOD GROUP SYSTEMS

- **Introduction**
- Blood group systems are any of the various classes into which human blood can be divided based on the specific antigens present on the surface of their red cells

- **Antigen**
- An antigen is any substance capable, under appropriate conditions, of inducing a specific immune response and of reacting with the products of that response

- **Blood group antigens**
- These are surface markers present on the red cell membranes, and are responsible for the identification of various blood group systems
- Though about 400 different blood group antigens exist, the antigens of the ABO and rhesus blood group system are the most clinically significant

- **ABO blood group system**
- Karl Landsteiner, an Austrian Scientist, described the ABO blood group system in 1901, when he discovered the A and B antigen on the surface of red cells
- The ABO blood group system is the most important in human blood transfusion

Blood group	Antigen on RBC	Antibody in serum
A	A	Anti-B
B	B	Anti-A
AB	A and B	None
O	None	Anti-A and Anti-B

- **Genetic basis of ABO system**
  - The ABO locus resides on chromosome 9 in human
  - The locus consists of three allelic genes: A, B and O
  - The A and B genes controls the synthesis of specific enzymes
  - The enzymes are responsible for the addition of single carbohydrate residue to H-substance
  - H-substance is a basic antigenic glycoprotein or glycolipid with a terminal L-fucose; on the surface of red cells
  - A-gene codes for the enzyme α 1-3-N acetyl galactosaminyl transferase that adds N-acetyl galactosamine to H-substance; forming the A-antigen
  - B-gene codes for the enzyme α 1-3 galactosyl transferase that add D-galactose to H-substance; forming the B-antigen
  - O-gene does not code for any enzyme; thus, does not transform the H-substance; and in turn has no detectable antigen (Amorphic)

- **Inheritance of ABO genes**
  - Inheritance of ABO genes follows the Mendelian fashion; with the A and B gene being co-dominant
  - The two genes an individual inherits from both parent (one from each) determines the individuals RBC antigens and in turn plasma antibodies

Gene from the parents	Genotype of offspring	Blood group of offspring
A + A	AA	A
A + O	AO	
B + B	BB	B
B + O	BO	
A + B	AB	AB
O + O	OO	O

- **Rhesus blood group system**
  - The rhesus blood group system was described by Landsteiner and Wiener; it was first discovered in a rhesus monkey; thus, the name "Rh factor"
  - The Rhesus blood group system (Rh system) is the most important after the ABO system in human blood transfusion

- **Genetic basis of Rhesus system**
  - The rhesus blood group system is one of the most polymorphic and immunogenic systems known in humans
  - At present, the Rh system consist of 50 antigens, among which 5 antigens: D, C, c, E, and e are important
  - Of all, the D antigen is the most important and is commonly called Rh-factor
  - The common terms Rh-positive or Rh-negative simply denotes the presence or absence of Rh-factor on the surface of an individual's RBCs
  - The Allele for the gene controlling the D-antigen is located on chromosome 1

Blood group system	Chromosome number	Association with transfusion reaction	Association with HDN
ABO	9	Yes (common)	Yes (usually mild)
Rhesus	1	Yes (common)	Yes
MNS	4	Yes (rare)	Yes (rare)
Duffy	1	Yes (occasional)	Yes (occasional)
Kidd	2	Yes (occasional)	Yes (occasional)
Kell	X	Yes (occasional)	Anemia not hemolysis
Lewis	19	Yes (rare)	No

- **Red cell Antibodies**
- **Anti-A and Anti-B antibodies**
  - These are naturally occurring antibodies to A and B antigens of the ABO system in the plasma of subjects lacking the corresponding antigen
  - They are usually immunoglobulin M, IgM; produced by plasma cells (B-lymphocytes)
  - They react optimally at cold temperature (4°C) and are thus, called cold antibodies
  - They are incapable of transplacental passage from mother to fetus

- **Anti-D antibodies**
  - Unlike in ABO system, the Rh system has no naturally occurring antibodies in plasma against the D-antigen
  - Antibodies are only developed in a Rh-negative individual following exposure to a Rh-positive blood
  - They are usually immunoglobulin G, IgG
  - They react optimally at warm temperature (37°C) and are thus, called warm antibodies
  - They are capable of passing from mother to fetus through the placental

CHAPTER 18: BLOOD TRANSFUSION AND ANTICOAGULANTS

- **Blood Transfusion**
- Blood transfusion is the safe transfer of whole blood or blood component from a donor directly into the blood stream of a recipient
- Transfusion of blood or blood component is without doubt an invaluable therapeutic measure; however, should not be given without an appropriate clinical indication, when the benefits outweigh its short and longer term risks.

- **Indications for blood transfusion**
- To restore blood volume following acute loss of >25 % of blood volume
- Major operations in which excessive blood loss is inevitable
- Severe anemia
- Patient with severe hemoglobinopathies e.g. sickle cell anemia, β-thalassemia major
- Patient requiring exchange blood transfusion

- **Criteria for blood donation**
- Donors should be between 18 - 65 years, with weight > 51kg
- Hemoglobin concentration should be > 13g/dl in males and > 12g/dl in females
- No major operation in the last 6 months
- No pregnancy within the last 12 months
- No blood donation in the past 4 months
- No blood transfusion within the past 12 months
- Donor should be free from the following:
  - Pregnancy or lactation
  - Cardiovascular diseases
  - Chronic renal disease

- Epilepsy and other CNS disorder
- Splenomegaly and hepatomegaly

— Donor should be free from history or clinical evidence of any of the following diseases:
- Chronic viral hepatitis (HBV and HCV)
- Syphilis
- Human immunodeficiency virus (HIV)
- Chaga's disease
- Human T-cell leukemia virus (HTLV)

- **Procedure of blood transfusion**

— A number of steps are taken to ensure that the recipient receives a compatible blood at the time of transfusion, these include:

- Blood collection from fit donors
- Blood storage at 2-6°C in sterile bags containing anticoagulants
- Grouping and cross matching of donor and recipient blood
- Administration and monitoring of the blood under strict asepsis

- **Grouping and cross matching**
— The ABO and Rh blood group of the patient is determined
— The donor blood is mixed with commercially-prepared antibodies against A, B, and D antigens i.e. anti-A, anti-B and anti-D antibody
— This is done in separate preparations for each of the antibodies, then observe for agglutination:

- If agglutination occurs: the donor blood reacts with that particular antibody and thus incompatible with blood containing that kind of antibody

- If agglutination does not: the donor blood does not have the antigens specific for that antibody and thus compatible with blood containing that kind of antibody

Donor blood group	Appropriate recipient
A	A and AB
B	B and AB
AB	AB
O	A, B, AB and O
Rh +ve	Rh +ve
Rh −ve	Rh +ve and Rh −ve

❖ ANTICOAGULANTS

— Anticoagulants are a class of drugs that work to prevent the coagulation of blood

▪ Classification

— Therapeutic anticoagulants
— Laboratory anticoagulants

● Therapeutic anticoagulants

— These are useful in in-vivo clinical therapy of thrombotic disorders in which an anticoagulant effect is desirable
— Examples are: Heparin, Warfarin

● Laboratory anticoagulants

— These are employed in routine hematological investigations and in blood banking procedures to maintain fluidity and viability of blood

- Examples: Ethylene diamine tetra-acetic acid (EDTA), Sodium citrate and heparin

- **Anticoagulants used in blood banking**
✓ **Acid citrate dextrose (ACD)**
- A solution of citric acid, sodium citrate and dextrose
- Citrate helps to chelate calcium
- Dextrose helps to improve RBC viability
- Blood can be stored up to 21 days with ACD

✓ **Citrate phosphate dextrose (CPD)**
- A solution of citric acid, sodium citrate, monobasic sodium phosphate and dextrose
- Citrate helps to chelate calcium
- Its slightly higher pH of 5.6 helps to preserve 2,3 DPG into the second week of storage
- Blood can be stored up to 28 days with CPD

✓ **Citrate phosphate dextrose adenine (CPDA)**
- A solution of CPD and adenine
- Adenine helps to stimulate ATP production by glycolysis; thus improving RBC survival
- Blood can be stored up to 28 days with CPDA

CHAPTER 19: BLOOD TRANSFUSION REACTIONS

– Blood transfusion reaction can be described simply, as the adverse effects of blood transfusion.

– The risks associated with the transfusion of any specific unit of blood are low if appropriate steps are taken.

– Blood transfusion reactions (BTR) can be conveniently divided into four:

- Acute non- immunologic BTR
- Acute immunologic BTR
- Delayed non immunologic BTR
- Delayed immunologic BTR

	Non- immunologic BTR	Immunologic BTR
Acute (<24hrs)	• acute sepsis or endotoxic shock (Bacteria) • Hypothermia • Hypocalcemia (in infants)	• Febrile non-hemolytic transfusion reactions • Acute hemolytic transfusion reactions • Allergic reactions (urticarial) • Anaphylactic reactions • TRALI (transfusion-related acute lung injury)
Delayed (>24hrs)	• HIV, Hepatitis C, Hepatitis B, CMV • Others: Parvovirus B19; hepatitis A; malaria; Chagas' disease; brucellosis; syphilis	• Delayed hemolytic transfusion reactions • Post-transfusion purpura (PTP) • Transfusion-associated graft-versus-host disease (TA-GvHD) • Immune modulation

❖ IMMUNOLOGIC BLOOD TRANSFUSION REACTION

▪ Acute hemolytic transfusion reactions

- This is the premature destruction of transfused red cells due to reactions with antibodies in the recipient serum
- The antibodies were formed as a result of previous exposure to similar antigens; through transfusions or pregnancies
- Such reactions may be immediately after the transfusion or delayed (2–3 weeks)
- The most severe reactions occur when a group O recipient is transfused with group A, B or AB red cells and less severe when group A red cells are transfused to a group B recipient, or vice versa
- Hemolysis may be intravascular (IgM) or extravascular (IgG)
- Intravascular haemolysis, is the most frequent and dangerous type of hemolytic transfusion reaction is associated with activation of the complement cascade by IgM antibodies, practically always due to ABO-incompatible blood transfusions
- Extravascular red cell destruction is mediated by IgG antibodies (e.g. of the rhesus system) and are generally less severe, as they are unable to activate the compliment cascade

● Clinical features
- Heat or pain in the cannulated vein
- headache
- Flushing
- Chest tightness
- Nausea and lumbar pain.
- Tachycardia
- Profound hypotension and collapse
- Rigors and pyrexia

- Jaundice and DIC
- Hemoglobinaemia, hemoglobinuria and hemosiderinuria
- Acute renal failure with oliguria and anuria

- **Management**
- Terminate the transfusion immediately
- Restore blood volume, and maintain blood pressure and urinary flow through fluid challenges and frusemide infusion
- Hydrocortisone 100mg intravenously and antihistamine may help to alleviate shock
- Appropriate blood component therapy will be required if there is DIC
- Renal team should be involved early if urine output is poor
- All packs of transfused units should be returned to the blood bank
- A sample should be sent for bacteriological testing and all urine passed during the first 24 hr should be measured and examined for Hb.
- Full blood count
- Direct antiglobulin test
- Urinalysis

- **Delayed hemolytic transfusion reactions**
- Reactions neither predictable nor preventable majority has been previously sensitized but the antibody is not detectable in routine pretransfusion testing
- transfusion of blood containing the antigens to which the recipient has been sensitized previously provokes a brisk

anamnestic response that is characteristic of the secondary immune response
- Within 5 to 10days, the antibody level rises and the transfused cells are removed from the circulation.

- **Clinical features**
- **The triad of :**
- fever
- hyperbilirubinaemia and
- anaemia

- **Treatment**
- if severely anaemic and needs transfusion; give blood that does not contain the offending antigen

- **Febrile transfusion reactions**
- Together with urticaria, these are the most common type of immunological reaction to blood transfusion
- Antibodies are directed usually against HLA antigens, or sometimes against granulocyte and more rarely to platelet-specific antigens; in a previously sensitized patient
- Onset is delayed until 30–90 min after the start of the transfusion

- **Clinical features**
- May solely be a rise in temperature
- Chills, headache or rigors may be present

- **Management**
- Slow the rate of transfusion

- Give antipyretic (e.g. paracetamol)
- Transfusion with buffy coat poor red cells and platelets should be tried
- Leucodepletion is also helpful

✓ Antihistamines are of no benefit

- **Transfusion-related acute lung injury (TRALI)**
- The reaction is due in most cases to passive transfer of leucoagglutinins in donor plasma (usually multiparous women), leading to endothelial and epithelial injury, alveolar damage and inflammatory
- Symptoms develop within 1–2 h, or up to 6 h after infusion

- **Clinical features**
- Pulmonary infiltrates on chest radiograph; accompanied by
- Fever and chills
- Cough and dyspnoea
- Low oxygen saturation
- Low or normal central venous pressure

- **Management: is essentially supportive, requiring high-dependency unit care, and careful attention to fluid balance.**

❖ NON-IMMUNOLOGIC BLOOD TRANSFUSION REACTION

- **Disease transmission**
- Reactions due to bacterial pyrogens in transfused blood may lead either to febrile reactions or to the far more serious manifestations of septic or endotoxic shock.

- Bacterial-transmitted infections are considerably more frequent than serious acute manifestations of virus-transmitted infections

- **Symptoms**
- High fever
- DIC with haemorrhagic phenomena
- shock and collapse

- **Diagnosis**
- Direct microscopic examination of the blood
- blood cultures from the recipient and the blood bag

- **Treatment**
- broad-spectrum intravenous antibiotics
- treatment of shock.

- **Prevention**
- stringent observation of procedures for aseptic techniques in blood collection and in the manufacture of anticoagulant solutions and packs.
- Blood should always be kept 2–6°C, and a unit of blood should never be removed and taken to the ward or theatre until it is required

- **Circulatory overload**
- This may occur in pregnant patients, patients with severe anaemia, and the elderly with compromised cardiovascular function

- Such patients will not tolerate the increase in plasma volume, and acute pulmonary oedema may develop.
- Thus in this category of patients, concentrated red cells should be given more slowly over 4 hrs and should be observed carefully for early signs of cardiac failure

- **Treatment**
- Discontinue the transfusion
- Propped the patient upright and give intravenous diuretics

- **Massive Transfusion**
- Massive transfusion is usually defined as the replacement of the total blood volume within a 24-h period

- **Effects of massive transfusion**
- Replacement of the total blood volume will inevitably lead to some dilution of platelets, as stored blood effectively has no functional platelets after 48 hrs
- Once 8–10 units of blood have been given to an adult, thrombocytopenia will usually be seen
- Coagulation factors will also be diluted as stored blood is administered

- **Clinical features:** low pH (acidosis), hypothermia, coagulopathy

- **Treatment:** FFP, cryoprecipitate

SECTION V   HEMATOLOGICAL MALIGNANCIES

CHAPTER 20: INTRODUCTION TO HEMATOLOGICAL MALIGNANCIES

- **Introduction**
- Hematological malignancies are clonal diseases that derive from a single cell in the bone marrow or peripheral lymphoid tissue that has undergone a genetic alteration
- They account for 8 - 9% of all malignant diseases

- **Classification**
- The world health organisation (WHO) in 2001 classified hematological malignancies into 3 broad groups:
- **Leukemias (30%)**
    - Acute lymphoblastic leukemia (ALL)
    - Acute myelogenous leukemia (AML)
    - Chronic lymphocytic leukemia (CLL)
    - Chronic myelogenous leukemia (CLL)
    - Acute monocytic leukemia (AMoL)

- **Lymphomas (56%)**
    - Hodgkin's lymphoma
    - Non-Hodgkin's lymphoma

- **Myelomas (14%)**

- **Classification of Cytotoxic Drugs**

Alkylating Agents	Cytotoxic antibiotics
Cyclophosphamide	Anthracyclines (e.g.
Chlorambucil	daunorubicin)
Busulfan	Hydroxodaunorubicin
Nitrogen mustard	(Adriamycin)

Melphalan	Mitoxantrone
Cisplatin	Idarubicin
	Bleomycin
Antimetabolites	**Plant derivatives**
Methotrexate	Vincrisinle (Oncovin)
6-Mercaptopurine	Vinblastine
6-Thioguanine	Epipodophyllotoxin (etoposide,
Cytosine Arabinoside	VP-16)

- Side effects of common cytotoxic drugs

Cytotoxic drug	Side effect
Cyclophosphamide	Hemorrhagic cystitis, cardiomyopathy, hair loss
Chlorambucil	Marrow aplasia, hepatotoxicity, dermatitis
Cisplatin	Renal dysfunction, neurotoxicity, ototoxicity
Methotrexate	Mouth ulcers, gut toxicity
Vincristine (Oncovin)	Neuropathy (Peripheral, bladder and gut)
Fludarabine	Immunosuppression, renal and neurotoxicity
Hydroxyurea	Pigmentation, nail dystrophy, skin ulceration

CHAPTER 21: ACUTE LEUKEMIAS

- **Introduction to Leukemias**
- Leukemias are a group of disorders characterised by accumulation of malignant white cells in the bone marrow and blood
- It may involve any cell line of the bone marrow or a stem cell common to several cell lines of the bone marrow

- **Classification**
- Leukemias are classified into two main groups:
  - Acute leukemias
  - Chronic leukemias

❖ **ACUTE LEUKEMIAS**
- By definition, acute leukemia is the presence of > 20% of blasts cells in the bone marrow at clinical presentation
- Blast cells, also called blasts or precursor cells, are any of the immature cells in the bone marrow e.g. myeloblasts, lymphoblasts, erythroblasts etc.

- **Characteristics acute leukemias**
- Onset is usually rapid
- It is very aggressive
- There is maturation arrest; thus, blast cells predominate
- Rapidly fatal if untreated
- Cure is achievable

- **Etiology of Acute Leukemias**
- **Unknown: in most cases**
- **Environmental agents**
- ✓ **Ionizing radiation**
- Especially among the survivors of the Hiroshima and Nagasaki atomic bomb in Japan

- People living in vicinity of ionizing radiation or high tension cables

✓ **Chemical carcinogens**
- Benzene and other petroleum products

- **Cytotoxic drugs**
- Alkylating agents – e.g. nitrogen mustard, chlorambucil, lomustine
- Topoisomerase II inhibitors – e.g. Etoposide, anthracyclines

- **Genetic or constitutional conditions**
- Down's syndrome – AML and ALL
- Bloom's syndrome - AML and ALL
- Fanconi's anemia - AML especially
- Ataxia telangiectasia – ALL and lymphomas

- **Pre-existing diseases**
- Aplastic anemia – ALL
- Paroxysmal nocturnal hemoglobinuria – AML, rarely ALL
- Myelodysplasia – AML
- Chronic myeloproliferative disorder - AML

- **Classification of acute leukemias**
- Based on the prominent blast cells involved in the expansion, acute leukemias are divided into two:
    - Acute lymphoblastic leukemia (ALL)
    - Acute myeloblastic leukemia (AML)

❖ ACUTE LYMPHOBLASTIC LEUKEMIAS (ALL)

- ALL is a malignant tumor of hemopoietic precursor cells of the lymphoid lineage, characterised by the accumulation of lymphoblasts in bone marrow and blood

▪ **Incidence of ALL**

- It is the most common form of leukemia in children
- Most cases occur between 3 to 7 years, falling off by age 10, with a second rise after age 40

▪ **Classification of ALL**

- Though several classification criteria are available for ALL, we would limit ourselves to the French-American-British (FAB) group classification:

● **FAB classification of ALL**

- Based on their studies on the morphology of blast cells, the French-American-British (FAB) groups have classified ALL into 3 subtypes:

✓ **L_1**
- Blast cells are small and uniform in size
- High nucleo-cytoplasmic ratio and scanty cytoplasm

✓ **L_2**
- Blast cells are large and heterogeneous
- Low nucleo-cytoplasmic ratio,
- with more prominent nucleoli

✓ **L_3**
- Presence of Burkitt type cells
- Large blast cells with vacuolated and strongly basophilic cytoplasm
- With prominent nucleoli

- L_1 is the subtype seen in about 80% of childhood ALL and the prognosis is good
- L_2 is the subtype seen in most adult cases and the prognosis is poor
- L_3 is the least common of the subtypes and the prognosis is very poor

❖ ACUTE MYELOBLASTIC LEUKEMIA (AML)

- AML is a malignant tumor of hemopoietic precursor cells of the non-lymphoid lineage, characterised by the accumulation of myeloblasts in bone marrow and blood

▪ Incidence of AML

- It occurs in all age groups
- It constitute only 10 – 15% of childhood leukemia
- Its incidence increases with age and thus the commoner form of acute leukemia in adults

▪ Classification of AML

- Though several classification criteria are available for AML, we would limit ourselves to the French-American-British (FAB) group and the WHO classification:

▪ FAB classification of AML

- Based on their studies on the morphology of blast cells, the FAB groups classified AML into 8 subtypes ($M_0 - M_7$):

- M_0 – undifferentiated myeloblastic cells
- M_1 – myeloblastic cells without maturation
- M_2 – myeloblastic cells granulocytic maturation
- M_3 – acute promyelocytic leukemia

- M_4 – myelomonoblastic cells with both granulocytic and monocytic maturation
- M_5 – acute monoblastic leukemia (M_{5A}) and acute monocytic leukemia (M_{5B})
- M_6 – erythroleukemia a.k.a. Di Guglielmo's disease
- M_7 – acute megakaryoblastic leukemia

- **WHO classification of AML**
- AML minimally differentiated
- AML without maturation
- AML with maturation
- Acute myelomonocytic leukaemia
- Acute monocytic leukaemia
- Acute erythroid leukaemia
- Acute megakaryocytic leukaemia
- Acute basophilic leukaemia
- Acute panmyelosis with myelofiborisis

- **Clinical features**
- The clinical features of acute leukemias are usually secondary to two broad pathological mechanisms:
- Bone marrow failure
- Organ infiltration

- **Bone marrow failure**
- Bone marrow failure is characterised by pancytopenia i.e. pronounced reduction in the number of erythrocytes, leukocyte, and platelets in the circulating blood.

✓ **Due to anemia:** pallor, lethargy, dyspnea
✓ **Due to neutropenia:** fever, malaise, features of mouth, throat, skin respiratory, perianal or other infections

✓ **Due to thrombocytopenia:** purpura, spontaneous bruise, bleeding gum, menorrhagia

- **Organ infiltration**
  - Bone tenderness
  - Lymphadenopathy (especially in ALL; rarely in AML)
  - Splenomegaly (moderate)
  - Hepatomegaly
  - Meningeal syndrome (characterised by; headache, nausea, vomiting, blurring of vision and diplopia)
  - Papilledema and at times hemorrhage
  - Testicular swelling
  - Mediastinal compression (in T-ALL)

- **Laboratory findings**
- **Full blood count**
  - Normocytic normochromic anemia
  - Thrombocytopenia
  - Total WBC count may be decreased, normal or increased

- **Peripheral blood smear: shows variable number of blast cells**
- **Bone marrow studies**
  - Hypercellular with > 20% leukemic blasts (diagnostic)
  - 10-40% of myeloblasts contain Auer rods (pathognomonic of AML)
  - Auer rods is never found in lymphoblasts or lymphocyte

- **Lumbar puncture (CSF examination)**
  - Increased spinal fluid pressure and contains leukemic cells

- **Biochemical tests**
  - Serum uric acid (increase)

- Serum lactate dehydrogenase (increased)
- Serum calcium (increased; though less common)

- **Radiology**
- Chest X-ray - Mediastinal mass (due to enlarged thymus or lymph nodes; seen in T-ALL)
- Abdominal ultrasound – enlarged para-aortic and other abdominal lymph nodes

- **Treatment**
- Supportive therapy
- Specific therapy

- **Supportive therapy**
- ✓ **Insert a central venous catheter**
- Hickman catheter is inserted into a central vein
- Serves as easy route of administration of chemotherapy, blood products, antibiotics etc.

✓ **Prevention of tumor lysis syndrome (TLS)**
- TLS is a combination of hyperkalemia, hyperuricemia, hyperphosphatemia and hypocalcemia due to rapid destruction of tumor cells
- It is prevented by administering: allopurinol, adequate intravenous fluid, alkalinisation of urine, rasburicase

✓ **Prevention of vomiting**
- Anti-emetic drugs e.g. metoclopromide, ondansetron, prochloperazine etc. are use in preventing nausea and vomiting

- **Prophylaxis and treatment of infection**
- Oral non-absorbable antibiotics for gut bacteria – neomycin and colistin
- Oral antibiotics – ciprofloxacin and co-trimoxazole
- Antifungal agents – Amphotericin B and fluconazole

✓ **Others**
- Blood product support
- Nutritional support
- Psychological support
- Pain management

- **Specific therapy**
- Administration of cytotoxic drugs (chemotherapy) is the mainstay of treatment in acute leukemia
- At least 3 cytotoxic drugs are combined; this is to increase cytotoxic effect, improve rate of remission and reduce drug resistance
- Administration of the drugs is done in cycles, this is to allow for regeneration of the damaged normal cells
- Chemotherapy in acute leukemia can be easily understood under the following headings:

- **Induction of remission**
- Remission is a valuable first step in the treatment of acute leukemias
- It is aimed at rapidly killing the tumor cells and getting the patient into a state of remission
- Remission is said to have occurred when:
    - < 5% blasts are found in the bone marrow
    - Peripheral blood count are normal

- No other symptom or sign of the disease is present

ALL	AML
• Dexamethasone • Vincristine • Asparaginase	• Cytosine arabinoside • Daunorubicin • Idarubicin • Mitoxantrone • 6-thioguanine • Etoposide

– Patients who fail to achieve remission have a poor prognosis

- **Intensification (consolidation)**
– Following remission, practically all patients will relapse without further chemotherapy; thus the need for intensification
– Intensification is aimed at eliminating the residual blast cells, using high doses of multi-drug chemotherapy
– The doses required are near the limit of the patients tolerability, thus a great deal of support is needed

– The following are drugs used in intensification: Vincristine, cyclophosphamide, cytosine arabinoside, daunorubicin, etoposide, 6-thioguanine, mercaptopurine

– They are used as blocks in different combinations

- **Maintenance**
– This is the extended use of multi-drug chemotherapy (for about 2 years) with the aim of achieving greater cell kill and reduced chance of relapse
– Maintenance is of greater relevance in ALL than AML (except in AML M_3)
– The drugs are used in maintenance in ALL and AML M_3:

ALL	AML M$_3$
Mercaptopurine	All trans-retinoic acid (ATRA)
Methotrexate	Mercaptopurine
Vincristine	Methotrexate
Prednisolone/Dexamethasone	

- **Central nervous system (CNS) directed therapy**
- ALL has a greater predilection for the CNS than AML; thus CNS therapy is relevant only in ALL
- As few of the systemically administered drugs is able to reach the cerebrospinal fluid, specific CNS treatment is required, and options include:

  - High dose methotrexate given intravenously
  - Intrathecal methotrexate or cytosine arabinoside
  - Cranial irradiation (should be avoided in children)

CHAPTER 22: CHRONIC LEUKEMIAS

- **Introduction**
- Chronic leukemia is an abnormal increase in white blood cell count due to malignant transformation of their progenitor cells

- **Characteristics chronic leukemias**
- Onset is insidious
- It is usually less aggressive
- maturation is unaffected; thus, lymphocytes predominate
- Not rapidly fatal, as disease progression is slow
- Cure is almost impossible to achievable

- **Classification of chronic leukemias**

Depending on the bone marrow cell line affected, chronic leukemias are broadly classified into 2 groups:

- Chronic myeloid leukemia (CML)
- Chronic lymphoid leukemia (CLL)

- ❖ **CHRONIC MYELOID LEUKEMIA (CML)**
- By definition; CML is a myeloproliferative disorder characterised by increased proliferation of the granulocytic cell line, without loss of their capacity to differentiate
- CML is also called chronic granulocytic leukemia, as it typically presents with increased granulocyte and immature precursor cell in the blood and bone marrow

- **Epidemiology**
- CML accounts for 15% of all leukemias
- It may occur at any age but most common between ages 40 and 60

- Annual incidence is 1.6/100,000
- Slightly commoner in males; with a ratio of 1.4 to 1
- It is the commoner form of childhood chronic leukemia

- **Predisposing factor**
- Though in most cases there are no predisposing factors identifiable, increased incidence has been associated with:
  - Heavy radiation exposure
  - Cigarette smoking

- **Genetic basis**
- The Philadelphia (Ph) chromosome has been identified as the pathognomonic mutation in CML
- Normally, the ABL gene, a proto-oncogen, lies on the long arm of chromosome 9; while the BCR gene lie on the long arm of chromosome 22
- Ph chromosome arise due to the translocation between chromosome 9 and 22; t(9;22)(q34;q11) during which the BCR-ABL fusion gene is formed

- **Pathogenesis**
- The resulting BCR-ABL fusion gene (an oncogene) codes for an abnormal fusion protein (an oncoprotein)
- The fusion protein has a molecular weight of 210 KDa, and thus, excess tyrosine kinase activity, as opposed to the normal protein with molecular weight of 145 KDa
- Following formation of the oncoprotein, it functions as a constitutively active tyrosine kinase that can phosphorylate a number of cytoplasmic substrates
- This feature, along with others leads to alteration in the cell proliferation, differentiation and survival

- **Clinical features**
- CML is often an incidental finding on routine blood examination or during investigation for unrelated disorders
- Symptoms when present may include:

Features of hypermetabolism	Weight loss, Lassitude, Anorexia Night sweat, Gout /renal impairment
Features of marrow failure	Infection, Fever, Generalized body pain, Neutropenia
Features of anemia	Pallor, Weakness, Dyspnea Intermittent claudication
Features of massive splenomegaly	Early satiety, Severe pain and discomfort in the splenic area
Features of thrombocytopenia	Bruising, Epistaxis, Petechiae and menorrhagia

- **Phases: Chronic phase, Accelerated phase, and Blast phase**
- **Chronic phase: In the chronic phase of CML, fewer than 10% of the cells in blood and bone marrow are blast cells**
- **Accelerated phase: here, 10 - 19% of the cells in blood and bone marrow are blast cells**
- **Blastic phase**
- In the blastic phase of CML, 20% or more of the cells in blood and bone marrow are blast cells
- If tiredness, fever, and splenomegaly occur during this phase, it is called blast crisis

- **Laboratory Findings**
- **Full blood count**
- Leukocytosis – usually > 50 x 10^9/L and at times >500 x 10^9/L
- Basophilia
- Platelet count is usually increased (though may be normal or decreased)

- Peripheral blood smear: normochromic normocytic anemia
- Bone marrow aspiration and cytology: definitive diagnosis for CML
- Biochemical tests: neutrophil alkaline phosphatase activity (low)

- Treatment
- First-line drugs
✓ Imatinib mesylate (Glivec)
  - A specific inhibitor of BCR-ABL fusion protein tyrosine kinase activity
  - At a dose of 400mg it is able to produce a complete hematological response in virtually all patients
  - Complete cytogenetic response; defined as the absence of Ph-positive metaphases on cytogenetic analysis of the bone marrow, is also achievable

✓ **Allopurinol**
  - Used in the initial phase of treatment to prevent hyperuricemia and gout

- **Second-line drugs**
  - Used in patients unable to take Imatinib or have poor response to it; they include:

✓ **Hydroxyurea**
  - It can control and maintain the WBC count in the chronic phase; however, it usually needs to be given indefinitely

✓ **Busulfan (Myleran)**
  - An alkylating agent

- It is also effective but has considerable long-term side-effects and thus reserved for patients not able to tolerate hydroxyurea

- α-interferon
- Stem cell transplantation

❖ CHRONIC LYMPHOID LEUKEMIA (CLL)

- By definition; CLL is a lymphoproliferative disorder characterised by clonal expansion and progressive accumulation of mature, but immunologically dysfunctional lymphocytes
- The CLL cells, which are monoclonal B-lymphocytes, typically accumulate in the blood, bone marrow and lymphoid tissues as a result of their prolonged life-span
- They are unique in being CD5+ andCD23+

- **Epidemiology**
- CLL is the most frequent type of leukemia in most part of world; however, it is rare in the far east
- It is a disease of the elderly, and the peak age of incidence is between 60 and 80 years
- Male to female ration is 2 to 1
- Unlike in other forms of leukemia, incidence is independent of radiation or chemical exposure
- However, there is a strong familial predisposition, as there is a 7-fold increased risk of the disease in close relatives of the patient

- **Genetic basis**
- Unlike in CML where the Ph chromosome is characteristic, there is no specific chromosomal anomaly typical of CLL
- Recent studies however have demonstrated several recurring chromosomal translocations that may be of both pathogenetic and prognostic significance.
- The most common of such clonal abnormality was
  - trisomy 12; others are:
  - Deletion of 13q14
  - Deletions at 11q23
  - Structural abnormalities of 17p involving P53 gene

- It suffix to mention that, defect in apoptosis typifies CLL, with majority of the cells being long-lived and out of the cell cycle i.e. in Go phase
- Thus, a small fraction of the cells replicating is responsible for their progressive accumulation

- **Etiology**
- Etiology of CLL is largely unknown

- **Risk Factors**
- Family history of CLL
- Family history of other lymphoproliferative diseases
- Bearing of the implicated chromosomal anomalies

- **Clinical features**
- About 50% of patient with CLL are asymptomatic at diagnosis; it is often an incidental finding on routine blood examination
- Symptoms when present may include:

✓ **Lymphadenopathy**
- This is the most frequent clinical sign

– Non-tender, discrete, symmetrical enlargement of cervical, axillary, or inguinal lymph nodes

✓ Immunosuppression
– a significant problem in them
– Caused by hypogammaglobulinemia and cellular immune dysfunction
– Infection is initially bacterial, but later viral and fungal

✓ Features of anemia and thrombocytopenia are often present
✓ Splenomegaly
✓ Hepatomegaly (less common, except in later stages)
✓ Tonsillar may be a feature

▪ **Laboratory findings**
● **Full blood count**
– Lymphocytosis - usually > 5 x 10^9/L and may be up to >300 x 10^9/L

● **Peripheral blood smear**
– 70-90% of the WBCs appear as small lymphocytes
– Smudge or smear cells (disrupted leukocytes) are also present
– Normocytic normochromic anemia (seen in later stage)
– Thrombocytopenia (in many patients)

● **Immunophenotyping**
– Shows the abnormal cells as B-cells (CD 19+) weakly expressing IgM or IgD
– Characteristically the cells are also CD5+ and CD23+ but CD79b- .

- **Bone marrow aspiration**
- Shows lymphocytic replacement of normal marrow elements

- **Immunological studies**
- Autoimmune hemolytic anemia is most frequently seen
- Immune thrombocytopenia, neutropenia and red cell aplasia are also seen

- **Treatment**
- Cures are rare in CLL; thus approach to therapy is conservative, aiming at symptom control, rather than at normal blood count
- Treatment options include:

- **Chemotherapy**
- Chlorambucil
- Purine analogues e.g. Fludarabine
- Monoclonal antibodies e.g. campath-1H (anti-CD52)
- Corticosteroids
- Ciclosporin

- Radiotherapy
- Splenectomy
- Immunoglobulin replacement
- Stem cell transplantation

CHAPTER 23 HODGKIN'S LYMPHOMAS

- **Introduction to Lymphomas**
- Lymphomas are any neoplastic disorder of the lymphoid tissue
- They are a group of diseases caused by malignant lymphocytes that accumulate in lymph nodes, causing the characteristic clinical features of lymphadenopathy

- **Types**
- Based on the histological presence of the neoplastic Reed-Sternberg (RS) cells, lymphomas are divided into two major types:

  - Hodgkin's lymphoma (RS cells are present)
  - Non-Hodgkin's lymphoma (RS cells are absent)

- ❖ **HODGKIN'S LYMPHOMA**
- This is the type of lymphoma characterised by presence of Reed-Sternberg (RS) cells in the diseased tissue

- **Cells found in Hodgkin's lymphoma**
- **Neoplastic cells**
- RS cells
- Mononuclear Hodgkin's cell

- RS cells are malignant, most often binucleated, giant histiocytes derived from a mutant B-cell
- The RS cells comprise only 1-2% of the total tumor mass
- Mononuclear Hodgkin's cell are found along with RS cells in Hodgkin's lymphoma; their fusion is believed to give the characteristic RS cells

- **Reactive cells**
- These are the infiltrating inflammatory cells (lymphocyte, eosinophils, plasma cells, neutrophils etc.) reacting to the ongoing neoplastic condition.

- **Incidence**
- Though it can present at any age, peak incidence is found among young adults
- It is rare among children
- Male to female ratio is 2 to 1

- **Pathogenesis**
- Little information exists on the pathogenesis of Hodgkin's lymphoma
- Immunoglobulin gene studies suggest that the RS cells are derived from a B-cell with a mutated immunoglobulin gene
- On account of the mutation, the abnormal B-cells acquired an increased rate of survival as they are able to escape apoptosis
- In addition, the cells are unable to synthesis a full-length immunoglobulin; thus are immunologically impotent
- Although Epstein-Barr virus (EBV) genome has been detected in >50% of cases in Hodgkin tissue, its role in the pathogenesis is not fully clear

- **Clinical features**
- **Lymphadenopathy**
- Painless, asymmetrical, rubbery enlargement of the superficial lymph nodes; involving the cervical, axillary, and inguinal lymph nodes
- Giving the bull-neck appearance

- **Splenomegaly and Hepatomegaly**
- The organomegaly are detectable clinically

- Splenomegaly occurs only in 50% of patients and not usually massive

- **Mediastinal involvement**
- Found in 6 – 11% of patient at presentation
- It is a feature of nodular sclerosing type, particularly in young women
- May be associated with pleural effusion or superior vena cava obstruction

- **Cutaneous Hodgkin's disease**
- A late complication in about 10% of patients
- Though unusual, other body organs e.g. bone marrow, gastrointestinal tract, lung CNS etc. may be involved

- **Constitutional symptoms**
- These are prominent in patient with wide spread disease; they include:
- Fever, Pruritus, Alcohol-induced pain, Weight loss, Profuse sweat (especially at night), Weakness, Anorexia

- **Laboratory findings**
- **Peripheral blood smear**
- Normochromic, normocytic anemia (most common)

- **Full blood count**
- Neutrophilia
- Eosinophilia (in one-third of patient)
- Lymphopenia and loss of cell-mediated immunity
- Platelet count is normal or increased in early disease and reduced in later stages

- **Other tests**
- Erythrocyte sedimentation rate (increased)

- C-reactive protein (increased)
- Serum lactate dehydrogenase (increased)

- **Diagnosis**
- The diagnosis of Hodgkin's is made by histological examination of an excised lymph node and demonstration of the characteristic RS cells
- The cells stain with CD30 and CD15 but negative for B-cell antigen expression

- **WHO/Histological classification**
- Histologically, the WHO classified Hodgkin's lymphoma into 5 types (four classic and one non-classic type)

- **Classic (shows RS cells)**
- Nodular sclerosis
- Mixed cellularity
- Lymphocyte rich
- Lymphocyte depleted

- **Non-classic (does not RS cells)**
- Nodular lymphocyte predominant

- **Ann Arbor staging of Hodgkin's lymphoma**
- **Stage I: node involvement in one lymph node area (either above or below the diaphragm)**
- **Stage II:** disease involving two or more lymph nodal areas confined to one side of the diaphragm.
- **Stage III:** disease involving lymph nodes above and below the diaphragm. Splenic disease is included here

- **Stage IV:** involvement outside the lymph node areas and to diffuse or disseminated disease in the bone marrow, liver and other extranodal sites.

✓ The stage number may be followed by the letter A or B to indicate the absence (A) or presence (B) of one or more of the constitutional features
✓ Also, the stage number may be followed by "S" to indicate splenic involvement e.g. IIIs

- Treatment
- **Patients with stage I and IIA:** radiotherapy alone

- **Patient with stage III and IV or stage I and II patient with bulky disease, type B symptoms or have relapsed**
- Cyclical chemotherapy is used; and the following combinations have been used:

✓ Adriamycin, bleomycin, vinblastine and dacarbazine (ABVD)
✓ Bleomycin, etoposide, doxorubicin, cyclophosphamide, Vincristine, procarbazine, prednisolone (BEACOPP)

CHAPTER 24: NON-HODGKIN'S LYMPHOMA (NHL)

- **Introduction**
- The term Non-Hodgkin's lymphoma encompasses a large and heterogeneous group of lymphoid tumors
- It involves the monoclonal proliferation and accumulation of lymphoid cells (usually B-cells) in lymph nodes and extranodal sites (bone marrow, spleen, liver and GI tract)

- **Peculiarities of NHL**
- It is commoner than Hodgkin's lymphoma
- Its clinical presentation and natural history are more variable than in HL
- Characterised by an irregular pattern of spread
- Significant portion of patient develop extranodal disease

- **Epidemiology**
- NHL is the most common hematological malignancy in the developed world; accounting for 5.4% of all cancers
- Though seen in all age groups, they are commoner among adults
- They are commoner among whites compared to blacks
- Male to female ratio is 2.6 to 1

- **Risk factors for NHL**
- In most cases, etiology of the disease is unknown, although infectious agents are important cause in particular subtypes.

Infectious Agent	Specific Organism	NHL Caused
VIRUSES	Human T-lymphotropic virus 1	Adult T-cell leukemia
	Epstein-Barr virus (EBV)	Endemic Burkitt's lymphoma Post transplant lymphoproliferative disease AIDS-related lymphoma
	Human herpes virus 8 (HHV-8)	Kaposi's sarcoma Primary effusion lymphoma
	Human immunodeficiency virus (HIV)	High-grade B-cell lymphoma
	Hepatitis C	Splenic marginal zone lymphoma
BACTERIA	Helicobacter pylori	Mucosal-associated lymphoid tissue (MALT) lymphoma
PROTOZOA	Malaria parasite	Endemic Burkitt's lymphoma

- **WHO histopathological classification of NHL**
- It suffix to know that NHL are otherwise known as B-cell and T-cell lymphoma
- B-cell disorder comprise about 85% of cases while T-cell and natural killer cell disorders account for the rest
- The cells involved in NHL be it B or T-cell may be either the precursor or mature cells
- With this background knowledge, understanding the WHO classification below should be easy.

Precursor B-cell neoplasm	Precursor T-cell neoplasms
B-lymphoblastic leukemia/lymphoma (precursor B-cell ALL, B-ALL/LBL)	T-cell lymphoblastic lymphoma/leukemia (T-ALL/LBL)
Mature B- cell neoplasms	**Mature T-cell and NK cell/neoplasms**
B-cell chronic lymphocytic leukemia/small	T-cell prolymphocytic leukemia T-cell granular lymphocytic

lymphocytic lymphoma	leukemia
B-cell prolymphocytic leukemia	Aggressive NK-cell leukaemia
Lymphoplasmacytic lymphoma	Adult T-cell lymphoma/leukemia
Splenic marginal zone B-cell lymphoma (+/-villous lymphocytes)	(HTLV-1+)
	Extranodal NK/T-celllymphoma, nasal type
Hairy cell Leukemia	Enteropathy-type T-cell lymphoma
Plasma cell myeloma/plasmacytoma	Mycosis fungoides/Sezary
Extranodal marginal zone B-cell lymphoma of	syndrome
MALT type	Anaplastic large cell lymphoma, primary cutaneous type
Mantle cell lymphoma	Peripheral T-cell lymphoma,
Follicular lymphoma	unspecified
Nodal marginal zone B-celllymphoma	Angioimmunoblastic T-cell
Diffuse large B-celllymphoma	lymphoma
Burkitt's lymphoma/Burkitt's cell leukaemia	Anaplastic large cell lymphoma, primary systemic type
Primary effusion lymphoma	
Mediastinal large B-cell lymphoma	

Table 24.2 ALL, acute lymphoblastic leukemia; HTLV, human T-cell leukemia/lymphoma virus; LBL, lymphoblastic lymphoma; MALT, mucosa-associated lymphoid tissue; NK, natural killer

- **Clinical subclassification of NHL**
– Based on their Clinical behaviour

Clinical type	Characteristics	Specific examples
Indolent/low-grade lymphoma	These lymphomas respond well to chemotherapy; however they are very difficult to cure	Follicular lymphoma (grade II) Lymphocytic lymphomas Lymphoplasmacytoid lymphoma Mantle cell lymphoma Marginal zone lymphomas
Aggressive/high-grade lymphoma	These lymphomas spread rapidly and needs urgent treatment; but are potentially curable with combination	Diffuse large B-cell lymphomas Burkitt's lymphoma Lymphoblastic lymphomas Adult T-cell lymphoma/leukemia

	chemotherapy	

- **Clinical features**
- **Superficial lymphadenopathy**
- Asymmetric, painless enlargement of nodes in one or more lymph node regions of; seen in most patient

- **Oropharyngeal involvement**
- Enlargement of oropharyngeal lymphoid structures making up the Waldeyers's ring
- Causes sore throat and noisy breathing

- **Abdominal involvement**
- Splenomegaly and hepatomegaly are often present
- Retroperitoneal and mesenteric lymph nodes are frequently involved

- **Constitutional symptoms**
- Fever (>38°C)
- Night sweats
- Weight loss (> 10% in the last 6 months)

- **Hematological features**
- Symptomatic anemia
- Neutropenia with infections
- Thrombocytopenia with purpura

- **Involvement of other organs**
- Skin, brain, testis and thyroid may but not frequently involved

- **Laboratory findings**
- **Lymph node biopsy for histology**
- This is the definitive investigation

- This is accompanied by immunophenotypic and genetic analysis
- B-cell expression of k or λ light chain confirms clonality

● **Hematological findings**

- Normochromic normocytic anemia is usual
- Autoimmune hemolytic anemia may occur
- Neutropenia and thrombocytopenia in advanced disease

● **Biochemical tests**

- Serum lactate dehydrogenase level (increase)
- Serum uric acid (increase)
- Immunoglobulin electrophoresis may reveal a paraprotein (β-microglobulin)

■ **Poor prognostic factors in NHL**

- Age > 60 years
- Number of extranodal site > 2
- Raised serum lactate dehydrogenase (LDH) level
- Raised β-microglobulin level
- Presence of constitutional symptoms
- Transformation from low to high-grade lymphoma

■ **Treatment**

NHL	Treatment
Follicular lymphoma	<ul><li>Radiotherapy **with**</li><li>Chlorambucil/cyclophosphamide, Vincristine, prednisolone (CVP) **or**</li><li>Fludarabine, Mitoxantrone, dexamethasone (FMD)</li></ul>
Lymphoplasmacytoid lymphoma	<ul><li>Oral chlorambucil, Fludarabine or rituximab</li></ul>
Mantle cell lymphoma	<ul><li>Chlorambucil/cyclophosphamide, Vincristine, prednisolone (CVP) **or**</li><li>Cyclophosphamide, hydroxodaunorubicin, Vincristine and prednisolone **with**</li></ul>

Marginal zone lymphoma	• Rituximab • Chemotherapy and/or radiotherapy with Rituximab • Patient with splenic MZL will benefit from splenectomy

❖ BURKITT'S LYMPHOMA (BL)

- **Burkitt Lymphoma:** is a highly aggressive B-cell non-Hodgkin lymphoma
- It is the fastest growing tumor known to man, with a doubling time of 24-36 hr, and a growth fraction of nearly 100%

- **Forms of BL**
- Endemic/African BL (eBL)
- Sporadic/Non-African BL (sBL)

	Endemic BL (eBL)	Sporadic BL (sBL)
Age	Younger children (4-7 yr)	Older children and young adults
Male : Female	2:1	2-3:1
Incidence	10/100,000	0.2-0.3/100,000
Geographical Distribution	Equatorial Africa, Papua New Guinea	Worldwide (especially North America and western Europe)
Common sites	Jaw, facial bones, abdomen	Abdomen, bone marrow, nasopharynx lymph nodes (LNs)
EBV Association	95% of eBL cases	15% of sBL cases
Chromosome 8 break point	Upstream of c-myc gene	Within c-myc gene

EBV: Epstein Barr Virus

- **Etiology and Pathophysiology**
- The exact mechanism by which BL develop is unknown, however,
- It is etiologically related to chronic Epstein-Barr virus (EBV) infection which, under the influence of persistent plasmodium falciparum infestation, causes reciprocal translocation of the *c-myc* **gene** on chromosome 8 to either:
- Immunoglobulin heavy chain region on chromosome 14 to give **t(8:14)(q24;q32)** (in > 80% of cases) or, in fewer cases, to
- Immunoglobulin kaplan light chain loci on chromosome 2 to give **t(8:2)** or
- Immunoglobulin lambda light chain loci on chromosome 22 to give **t(8:22)**
- This translocation thus triggers malignant transformation of the B-cells

- **Clinical features**
- ◆ **Jaw swelling**
- Most common presentation in eBL (i.e. in younger children)
- Swelling is painless and fast growing; may be unilateral or bilateral
- Maxilla is more commonly affected than the mandible
- Maxillary tumor may spread to involve the orbit (causing proptosis)
- May also cause loosening or loss of teeth, resulting in feeding and speech difficulty

- ◆ **Abdominal swelling**
- Most common presentation in sBL (i.e. in older children)

158

- Usually involves the ovaries, kidneys, mesenteric and retroperitoneal LNs
- May cause abdominal pain, abdominal distention and ascites

♦ **CNS Involvement**
- Intracranial BL may cause CN palsies (esp. **3** and **7**; others: 2,4,6,10), as well as raised intracranial pressure, headaches and visual impairment
- Extradural BL may compress the spinal cord to give flaccid paraplegia, as well as bowel (constipation) and bladder (incontinence) dysfunction

♦ **Others**
- sBL patients may present with dysphagia and airway obstruction from nasopharynx involvement or bowel obstruction from ileal-cecal intussusception
♦ **Constitutional (B) symptoms:** fever, weight loss, night sweats, fatigue

✓ **Other sites of BL:** breast, thyroid, parotids, testes, skin, lungs, spleen and liver.
- Involvement of these sites, though uncommon, is a poor prognostic sign

▪ **Staging**
- **Stage A:** single extra-abdominal tumor site
- **Stage AR:** intra-abdominal tumor, with > 90% of tumor resected

- **Stage B:** multiple extra-abdominal tumors
- **Stage C:** intra-abdominal tumor
- **Stage D:** intra-abdominal tumor with one or more extra-abdominal tumor

- **Investigations**
- **Specific**
- **Cytology (FNAC):** reveals **Burkitt cells** *(round non-cleaved B-cells with basophilic cytoplasm, fat filled vacuoles, and a nucleus containing multiple nucleoli)*
- **Histology:** shows **starry sky appearance** *(phagocytic macrophages, with pale foamy cytoplasm, scattered diffusely on a bluish background of closely apposed tumor cells)*

- **Supportive**
- **X-ray:** jaw (shows loss of lamina dura), chest (may show pleural effusion) etc
- **Other Imaging modalities *(for tumor extent and staging):*** USS, CT, MRI or PET scan of head, spine, chest, abdomen, pelvis etc.
- ◆ **FBC:** may reveal lymphocytosis or pancytopenia (if the bone marrow is involved)
- ◆ **LP:** may reveal increased CSF cell count (pleocytosis), reduced glucose level etc.

- ◆ **Chemistries**

- **E/U/Cr, calcium, phosphate and uric acid:** hyperkalemia, hyperphosphatemia, hyperuricemia and hypocalcemia may be present due to tumor lysis
- Uric acid nephropathy and oliguric renal failure may accompany tumor lysis, causing elevated urea and creatinine
- **Serum LDH:** almost always elevated in BL; used to monitor treatment response
- **B$_2$-microglobulin:** a predictor of extent of disease and a marker of early relapse

- **Treatment**
- **Supportive**
- This basically aims at preventing tumor lysis syndrome (TLS)
- TLS is a combination of **hyperkalemia, hyperuricemia, hyperphosphatemia** and **hypocalcemia** resulting from rapid destruction of tumor cells.

- **Adequate hydration:** with IV fluids, given 24 hr prior to chemotherapy
- **Rasburicase:** prevents hyperuricemia. (0.2 mg/kg IV daily for 5 days)
- **Allopurinol:** used to prevent hyperuricemia in lower risk patients and those who cannot tolerate rasburicase. (10 mg/kg/day PO in 3 divided doses)
- Alkalinisation of urine with sodium bicarbonate
- Frequent electrolyte monitoring
- ✓ **NB:** *allopurinol is a xanthine oxidase inhibitor while rasburicase is a recombinant urate oxidase*

- **Definitive**
- Intensive systemic chemotherapy is the mainstay of treatment of all stages of BL
- Treatment approaches currently available include:
- ✓ Modified Ziegler's Regimen
- ✓ CODOX-M/IVAC Regimen (Magrath Regimen)
- ✓ Hyper-CVAD Regimen
- ✓ Combination regimen followed by autologous stem cell transplantation (SCT)

- ◆ **Modified Ziegler's Regimen**
- With an interval of 2 wk in between, the patient receives 6 courses of:
  - IV cyclophosphamide: 1000 mg/m^2 on day 1
  - IV Vincristine (oncovin): 1.4 mg/m^2 on day 1
  - Methotrexate: 15 mg/m^2 on days 2 and 3
  - Tab Prednisolone: 40 mg/m^2 daily for 5 days

- **CNS prophylaxis:** intrathecal methotrexate (15 mg/m^2 on days 1 and 4) ± cytarabine and hydrocortisone

- ◆ **CODOX-M/IVAC Regimen (Magrath Regimen)**
- A shorter, more intensive, and highly effective regimen developed by Magrath
- It utilizes cyclophosphamide, vincristine, doxorubicin, high-dose methotrexate / ifosfamide, etoposide, and high-dose cytarabine

- ◆ **Hyper-CVAD Regimen**

- This involves use of modified fractionated cyclophosphamide, vincristine, doxorubicin, and dexamethasone

✓ **Rituximab**
- Rituximab is a recombinant antibody that targets CD20 on surface of B-cells
- It has been incorporated into most of the existing regimens, and has been proven to improve remission and overall survival

• **Monitoring**
- **Weekly FBC:** WBC should be ≥ 2000/uL (absolute neutrophil count ≥ 1000/uL), PCV ≥ 30%, platelet ≥ 100,000/uL.
- **Others:** E/U/Cr, liver function test, lactate dehydrogenase, B_2-microglobulin etc.

■ **Poor Prognostic Factors**
- CNS involvement
- Bone marrow involvement
- High tumor burden
- Age at presentation > 13 yr
- Male sex
- High serum LDH and uric acid

CHAPTER 25: OVERVIEW OF MYELOPROLIFERATIVE DISORDER

- Myeloproliferative disorders, now known as myeloproliferative neoplasms (MPN) are clonal diseases of single Pluripotent bone marrow stem cells
- They are characterised by proliferation of one or more myeloid cell lines with excessive accumulation of such cells

- **Genetic basis**
- Presence of acquired mutation of the Janus-associated kinase 2 (JAK-2) in the clonal cells
- There may also be deletion in long arm of chromosome 20; del(20q)

- **Risk factors**
- Exposure to radiation
- Exposure to industrial solvents e.g. benzene or toluene

- **Classification**
- Based on the presence or absence of the abnormal Philadelphia chromosome in the clonal cells, the WHO has classified MPN into two groups:
- Philadelphia chromosome positive (ph +ve)
- Philadelphia chromosome negative (ph -ve)

- **Philadelphia chromosome positive (ph +ve)**
- Chronic myeloid leukemia (CML)

- **Philadelphia chromosome negative (ph -ve)**
- This group is further subdivided into two, depending on whether the clonal cells are leukocytes or not:

- Leukemic
- Non-leukemia

Leukemic	Non-Leukemic
• Chronic neutrophilic leukemia (CNL) • Chronic eosinophilic leukemia (CEL) • Hypereosinophilic syndrome (HES)	• Polycythemia vera (PV) • Essential thrombocytopenia (ET) • Primary myelofibrosis (PMF) • Mastocytosis (MS) • Systemic Mastocytosis (SM) • Myeloproliferative neoplasm unclassified (MPN-u)

– Chronic myeloid leukemia (CML) was discussed in chapter … and polycythemia Vera (PV) is discussed in the next chapter

CHAPTER 26: POLYCYTHEMIA

- **Definition**
- Polycythemia also known as eryrhrocytosis is an increase in hemoglobin concentration of an individual above the upper limit of normal for his age, sex and race

- **Classification of Polycythemia**
- Absolute polycythemia
- Relative polycythemia

- **Absolute polycythemia**
- This is an actual increase in the red cell mass of the blood, caused by sustained overactivity of the erythroid component of the bone marrow
- It is further subdivided into:
  - Primary polycythemia (polycythemia rubra vera)
  - Secondary polycythemia

- **Relative polycythemia**
- The red cell mass of the blood is normal, but appears to be raised due to a decrease in the plasma volume
- It is a.k.a. pseudopolycythemia

- **Causes of relative polycythemia**
- Dehydration (water deprivation, vomiting)
- Stress
- Plasma loss (burns, enteropathy)
- Cigarette smoking

❖ **PRIMARY POLYCYTHEMIA (POLYCYTHEMIA RUBRA VERA)**
- PRV belongs to a class of disease called myeloproliferative disorders (Non-leukemic type)

- It is characterised by abnormal proliferation of all hematopoietic stem cells and an absolute increase in red cell mass and total blood volume

- **Genetics basis of PRV**
- The increase in red cell mass, typical of this disease, is due to clonal malignancy of a marrow stem cell
- Malignant transformation of the marrow stem cell follows the acquisition of JAK2 V617F somatic mutation, which gives it and its progeny a proliferative advantage over surrounding normal cells
- The JAK2 V617F somatic mutation is present in hemopoietic stem cells of almost 100% of affected individuals
- Chromosomal abnormalities such as; 9p or 20q are found in a minority of patient

- **Age and sex distribution of PRV**
- PRV is rare among children and young adults
- Median age of presentation is 50 – 60 years
- Sex incidence is equal

- **Clinical features of PRV**
- The clinical features of PRV are the result of hyperviscosity, hypervolemia, and hypermetabolism; they include:
- Recurrent headaches
- Dyspnoea
- Blurred vision
- Night sweat
- Pruritus (characteristically after a hot bath)
- Plethoric appearance:
    - ruddy cyanosis
    - conjuctival suffusion
    - retinal venous engorgement
- Hepatosplenomegaly (in 75% of patients)

- Thrombotic phenomena:
    - cerebrovascular disease
    - myocardial infarction
    - deep vein thrombosis
    - peripheral arterial occlusion

- Spontaneous bleeding:
    - epistaxis
    - ecchymosis
    - upper gastrointestinal bleeding

- Hypertension (in 1/3 of patient)
- Gout (due to increased uric acid production)
- Peptic ulceration (in 5- 10% of patients)

- **Diagnosis of PRV**
- **WHO criteria for diagnosis of PRV**
- ✓ Major criteria
- Hemoglobin concentration; >18.5g/dL in male and >16.5g/dL in female
- Red cell mass >25% above mean normal predicted value
- Presence of JAK-2 mutation

✓ **Minor criteria**
- Bone marrow trephine with trilineage proliferation
- Subnormal serum erythropoietin level
- Endogenous erythroid colony formation invitro

❖ *2 major and 1 minor criteria OR 1st major and 2nd minor criteria confirms the diagnosis of PRV*

- **Laboratory findings in PRV**
- **Full blood count**
  - PCV is increased
  - Red cell count is increased
  - Total red cell volume is increased
  - Neutophilic leukocytosis and increased circulating basophils
  - Platelet count is increased

- **Bone marrow analysis**
  - JAK2 V617F mutation is present in bone marrow and peripheral blood granulocytes in nearly 100% of patient
  - Bone marrow is hypercellular with prominent megakaryocyte (best assessed by a trephine biopsy)

- **Biochemical findings in PRV**
  - Neutrophil alkaline phosphatase (increase)
  - Serum erythropoietin (decrease)
  - Serum vitamin B12 (increase)
  - Expression of PRV-1; a surface receptor (increase)
  - Expression of c-mpl; thrombopoietin (decrease)
  - Plasma urate (increase)
  - Serum lactate dehydrogenase (normal)

- **Treatment**
  - Treatment of PRV is aimed at maintaining normal blood count
  - PCV should be maintained at 45%
  - Platelet count maintained below 400×10^9/L
  - Options of treatment include:

- **Venesection**
  - To reduce PCV below 45%
  - Indicated in younger patients and those with mild disease at the start of therapy

— However, this does not control platelet count

- **Cytotoxic myelosuppression**
— Considered in patient with poor tolerance to Venesection, symptomatic splenomegaly etc.
— Drugs include:
    • Hydroxycarbamide (hydroxyurea)
    • Busulfan
    • Pipobroman

— Phosphorus-32 therapy (in older patient with severe disease)
— Interferon
— Aspirin (to reduce thromboembolic complications)
— Anagrelide (reduces RBC producing cells)
— Melphalan (an Alkylating agent)
— JAK-2 inhibitors (ruxolitinib, tofacitinib)
— Allopurinol (for gout)
— Ranitidine (for pruritus)

❖ SECONDARY POLYCYTHEMIA
— This is caused by either natural or artificial increase the production of erythropoietin, causing an increased production of erythrocytes

- **Causes of secondary polycythemia**
— High altitude
— Chronic obstructive pulmonary disease (COPD)
— Cyanotic congenital heart disease
— Hydronephrosis
— Nephroblastoma

- Heavy cigarette smoking
- Uterine Leiomyoma
- Cerebellar hemangioblastoma
- Hepatocellular carcinoma
- Androgen abuse
- Gaisbock syndrome

- **Treatment**
- Treat the underlying cause

Thank you for reading! If you enjoyed this book or found it useful
I would be very grateful if you would post a short review on Amazon.
Your support really does make a difference and I read all the reviews personally so I can get your feedback and make this book even better.
Thank you!!!

Made in United States
Troutdale, OR
12/30/2024

27410900R10095